Setting Up New Services in the NHS

Community, Culture and Change
(formerly Therapeutic Communities)
Series editors: Rex Haigh and Jan Lees

Community, Culture and Change encompasses a wide range of ideas and theoretical models related to communities and cultures as a whole, embracing key Therapeutic Community concepts such as collective responsibility, citizenship and empowerment, as well as multidisciplinary ways of working and the social origins of distress. The ways in which our social and therapeutic worlds are changing are illustrated by the innovative and creative work described in these books.

other books in the series

Setting Up New Services in the NHS

'Just Add Water!'

Kingsley Norton

Community, Culture and Change 13

Jessica Kingsley Publishers
London and Philadelphia

First published in 2006
by Jessica Kingsley Publishers
116 Pentonville Road
London N1 9JB, UK
and
400 Market Street, Suite 400
Philadelphia, PA 19106, USA

www.jkp.com

Library of Congress Cataloging in Publication Data

Norton, Kingsley.
  Setting up new services in the NHS : 'just add water!' / Kingsley Norton.
    p. cm. -- (Community, culture, and change ; 13)
  Includes bibliographical references and index.
  ISBN-13: 978-1-84310-162-8 (pbk. : alk. paper)
  ISBN-10: 1-84310-162-9 (pbk. : alk. paper) 1. Henderson Hospital (Surrey, England)--Adminis-
tration. 2. Health planning--Great Britain. 3. National health services administration--Great Britain. I.
Title. II. Series.
  RA395.G6N68 2006
  362.10680941--dc22

                                                      2006011505

British Library Cataloguing in Publication Data
A CIP catalogue record for this book is available from the British Library

ISBN-13: 978 1 84310 162 8
ISBN-10: 1 84310 162 9

Printed and bound in Great Britain by
Athenaeum Press, Gateshead, Tyne and Wear

To S.L.

Contents

List of Tables and Figures

Preface

The 1990s saw massive organisational change within the NHS, including the separation of its 'purchasing' and 'providing' functions, these being devolved to separate authorities and distinct personnel in April 1991. Not obviously inconveniencing much of medical practice, nor many aspects of general psychiatry, some specialist (tertiary level) services were put at risk, such as the national personality disorder (PD) service at the Henderson Hospital in South West London. This was because 'out of area' referrals, i.e. those patients referred from further afield than the immediate local (purchasing) area, had to be funded individually on a 'cost per case' basis. At Henderson, two outcomes were commonly encountered. Either no funding was forthcoming or decisions to fund were delayed. According to Department of Health guidelines, such decisions should have been made within 48 hours. In our experience, decisions not only took weeks to be made but 34 per cent of such referrals were not funded (Dolan and Norton 1992).

Henderson, in theory, had to attempt to do business with up to 200 purchasers (the then district health authorities) across the UK. In practice, such a marketing task was impossibly large and PD clients did not usually compete well with other patients who needed such 'cost per case' funding. The result for Henderson was an untenable situation. On its own the local referral base could not guarantee sufficient patients to safeguard the clinical viability of its unusual treatment approach – a democratic 'therapeutic community' (TC). Henderson would need to close. With much support from inside and outside the TC world, however, a temporary 'regional' solution was identified, meaning that Henderson's future was secure at least for a while.

It was fortunate therefore that in 1994 an interdepartmental government report – the Reed Report – was published, detailing the needs of the so-called 'difficult and offender' patient group, part of which formed the staple diet of Henderson's TC (Reed 1994). One of the report's recommendations was that there should be 'more units such as the Henderson Hospital'. It was the effect of this document, together with Henderson's own lobbying of the Department of Health about the paucity of PD services, that led to the opportunity to bid to develop further units based on the democratic TC developed at Henderson. It was also Government policy to improve equity of access to specialist services across the country and to implement evidence-based practice within the field of healthcare.

On 7 June 1996, therefore, at a crucial meeting in the Department of Health, in the light of the Reed Report recommendations and these other factors (including an informal presentation of Henderson's evidence base), it was agreed that national funding for Henderson could be sought. However, as it was put to us, this could only be if there were 'Hendersons in the North, South, East and West'. In essence this meant Henderson Hospital (at the time part of the St Helier NHS Trust) finding suitable partner NHS Trusts with whom to collaborate to create further TCs. Together we could submit a joint bid to the Department by its deadline of November 1996. The Department of Health's gauntlet had been thrown down. Bravely or foolishly, we picked it up.

Unfortunately, the imminent arrival of the holiday season dictated that little activity took place till September. Then, geography figured in the decision as to whom to approach, as well as whether their service was part of a dedicated mental health Trust. Mental health services embedded in a 'general' Trust – physical medicine, surgery, etc. – were, we thought, unlikely to be able to invest sufficiently in such a replication project as ours, because of a lack of focus on and support for mental health. With these assumptions in mind, we contacted any relevant clinician known to us to be 'expert' in the PD field to see if they were interested in our potential project. The 'we' was mainly me, but I was supported tremendously by Henderson's marketing and information manager (Richard Bulmer) and researcher (Fiona Warren). Both were willing to rearrange their work schedules around mine to present a series of 'road-shows'. Subsequently, we exhibited our presentation to the interested parties. It included the research findings that had so impressed the Reed working group (and the Department of Health), together with details of the proposed project to develop further 'Hendersons'. In parallel, Fiona worked tirelessly to get the bid documentation into a presentable format that might stand a good chance of success, or at least of not being overlooked. The finished product weighed several pounds and was in an eye-catching box-file (no expense spared there). It contained, among other things, a book of Henderson's publications, masses of data describing and supporting the Henderson model and even a video of Henderson, which had been made by an ex-patient of the hospital – everything bar a Henderson T-shirt and kitchen sink. It would represent our third and final attempt to secure national funding, the effect of which would be to remove us and our clientele from the deleterious effect of the purchaser–provider split.

Early snags

Everyone we approached was interested – at least to know more about what was envisaged by our replication project. However, we had decided that we could only progress the enterprise on the basis of a thorough discussion with relevant Trust personnel – not only with the identified 'expert' but also with their multi-disciplinary and senior managerial colleagues. The 'road-shows' therefore needed to be well prepared and clearly presented for this wide audience to feel adequately informed. As we still had our day jobs to do, we were limited in how many presentations we could put on in the time available – effectively, just September and October 1996. This meant closing the list to some interested parties we had hoped to visit. We had to leave time to receive firm bids, to shortlist (if necessary) and to work together to finalise the documentation and submit it – by the end of November. Time was short. We presented to the North East, North West, West Midlands (in two places), Oxford and South West areas.

We became aware, all too painfully, that some esteemed colleagues had felt rejected and hurt by not having been approached. This had not been our intention. Rightly or wrongly, we had decided not to approach colleagues from other TCs. In part this strategy was borne out of a sense of modesty and our not wishing to impute that there might be something in their own TC approach that could be improved by adopting Henderson's particular 'democratic' model. (We might note in passing that Henderson's second failed bid for central funding had been a joint bid with the Cassel Hospital, whose therapeutic programme was established by Tom Main). Therefore, even before our bid had been submitted, the mere fact of a decision to bid, which was not a closely kept secret, was exerting a negative influence from unexpected sources – some of our TC colleagues. I received complaining telephone calls, lasting 45 minutes each, from two eminent TC figures! Henderson was in some way 'doing the dity', as one of them later eloquently summarised it. Their shared view was that the development of more TCs, Henderson's potential 'success', could only be at the expense of existing TCs. The ensuing events, recalled here, may tell a different story.

Success?

In 1996, ours was one of over 50 bids received by the National Specialist Commissions Advisory Group of the Department of Health. It was one of three psychiatric bids submitted. We had been led to believe by a senior civil servant involved that we would be likely to be informed (were we to be successful) towards the end of February but certainly by 28 March 1997. Well, the world does not revolve around Henderson Hospital, or so we were soon to learn. The Department of Health requested more information in support of our bid, but not all at once. To do so might have truncated the process. No, first, we were asked to provide more detail to show how we could set up four severe PD services in three years. Then, in May 1997, we were asked how we would go about setting up just three, then just two and then just one new 'Henderson'. This requirement, repeatedly to re-work the plans, was very time-consuming(and irritating). We still had not given up our day jobs. But we were committed – probably certifiable – so we complied. In late October 1997, we heard that we had been successful and were contracted to set up two new services based on the Henderson model. None involved in the Henderson replication project believed that it would be easy. We knew that there was no simple recipe to follow.

As the reader will discern, this book reflects my own particular perspective on the project, hence it is a subjective account. I therefore apologise in advance if any of those people mentioned or left out feel aggrieved thereby or believe that I have knowingly misrepresented either the matters discussed or the intentions of those also involved. I have attempted to present the facts and situations as I saw them. Much of the information contained is derived from contemporaneous notes or the minutes of meetings agreed by all involved. The project is the largest and most fulfilling of my professional career, and my hope is that some of what I have learnt can be passed on to others who are attempting to set up new NHS services.

The books falls into three parts. Part I comprises Chapters 1 and 2 and spans the period July 1997 to September 2000. In Chapter 1 the scene is set for the replication project through a description of Henderson Hospital's history and the relevance of this for its integral organisation ('structure') and ideology (part of its 'culture'). The structural elements are considered in relation to the clinical difficulties posed in treating clients with severe personality disorder in a specialist inpatient setting. The aim is to enable the reader to understand the nature and complexity of the therapeutic system to be replicated. In this way the size of the replication task can be appreciated. Chapter 2 reveals how we distilled our own understanding of the clinical workings of the democratic therapeutic community, in order for it to be rendered digestible to the staff in the new services. The aptly named Henderson Development Team (HDT) was set up to create, deliver and evaluate the training programme for new staff, and to this end we formed a close collaboration with former service users of the Henderson – the 'Volunteers'. This approach reflected the ideology of the service, which requires particularly close working relationships not only between staff but with our clients – 'communalism' (Rapoport 1960). The chapter also describes how the first two phases of the training of new staff were implemented.

Part II comprises Chapters 3–5 and covers particularly the period from September 2000 to March 2002 – the first 18 months of operation of the newly set up services. Chapter 3 describes in detail the early visits of HDT to the new services during the first six months after opening – the third phase of new staff training. Chapter 4, deriving from diary entries, reports on the difficulties encountered during the first months of operation of the new therapeutic communities, in pursuing the goal of replication. Chapter 5, starting from the inception of the collaboration, provides a retrospective analysis of how such difficulties might have arisen.

Part III covers, in overview, the whole period of the replication project. Chapter 6 provides a summary of the independent researchers' findings with respect to replication, including their conclusions. Chapter 7 is my evaluation of the aftermath of the replication process. In Chapter 8, I attempt to draw lessons from this project that might be applicable more generally to others in the NHS.

Acknowledgements

I need to thank so many people for the part they played, directly and indirectly, in the production of this book. It is invidious to place people in order of my indebtedness to them but necessary in any list of those to be acknowledged if only for reasons of legibility. The mind boggles at what such a list piled high upon itself might look like and how difficult to decipher.

My thanks go to those who made the replication project possible in the first instance. A range of civil servants were persuaded by Henderson's evidence base and believed its service could be a model for other personality disorder services. However, my particular thanks go to Dr Dilys Jones and Dr Sheila Adam. Dame Fiona Caldicott, as former President of the Royal College of Psychiatrists and Consultant Psychotherapist, presented our case to the National Specialist Commissioning Group (NSCAG). My sincere thanks therefore go to her for her confidence in our democratic therapeutic community (TC) model and its promising evidence base, as well as for her excellent communication skills. I thank NSCAG for accepting the challenge to support our bid, the first one to set up new highly specialist services at a distance, albeit they did so nervously.

The various Trusts involved with the replication are to be thanked. Their names changed during the course of the project but in particular I wish to thank the three original Chief Executives – Nigel Sewell (St Helier NHS Trust), Sue Turner (who took on the mantle only days into her post in South Birmingham) and Peter Clarke (Salford) – for their support. In their own ways the successive Trusts often travelled alongside us during the bumpy ride of this project, though not as much as we would have liked at certain points. The Chairman of St Helier Trust, Sir Jeremy Elwes, was always most encouraging of Henderson's work and its replication mission.

Staff in the parent Henderson did most of the difficult and non-exotic work of keeping the service going. Those of us involved in recruiting and training new staff and getting the new services off the ground had the more glamorous parts to play. Here I especially thank Richard Bulmer and Fiona Warren for their unflagging support from the very start of the project; without them there would have been no bid and hence no project and no new TCs. Dr Jan Birtle and Dr Keith Hyde, Directors of the new services, merit my praise as well as thanks for picking up the respective gauntlets and striving so valiantly and successfully in setting up their TC-based services. The three of us went through a lot together and came out the other side not only respecting but also valuing one another's personal commitment, professionalism and clinical skills.

The importance of the role of residents and ex-residents – the 'Volunteers' – in the collaborative replication endeavour cannot be exaggerated. To them I owe a particular debt of gratitude for their untiring efforts, highly relevant expertise and consistent valuing of the project. Time and again they held the more sensible views and were the saner voices, which were consequently more influential, and listened to by staff and residents in the new services. Indeed, this book is dedicated to the memory of one Henderson ex-resident who contributed to the replication task though was unable to sustain sufficient investment in herself to see the fruit of her own and others' labour in respect of this project.

I must thank the High Security Psychiatric Services Commissioning Board (superseded by the Forensic Mental Health Research and Development Programme) for providing the funding for the research to test whether replication had been achieved. Although they supported the relevant work, some of which is contained in this book, all of the views expressed are mine and not necessarily those of the Programme or the Department of Health. I am most grateful to the diligence and resilience of the research team and of its supervisory group who brought welcomed sanity, as well as intellectual rigour and method, to the research aspect of the project. Like the replication exercise itself, much of the research did not turn out to be straightforward. Susan Ormrod bore the brunt of the early difficulties and was frequently alone in the field for long periods in the early days!

Many secretarial staff from Henderson and St George's contributed to the production of this book, through correcting my own typed efforts and revamping figures, tables and appendices. I thank you all but especially Sue Garner. She managed to keep tabs on the many different drafts of the various chapters, when I was being my usual disorganised and technophobic self. The editors and publishers I also thank for their invitation to add to their excellent series of texts in the field of TCs and for their patience in my not completing mine on time. The delays caused by the unexpected need to focus my efforts again on keeping Henderson open (as far as this was in my control) were of others' making. However, these also provided me with more piquant material for the final literary product. There should be a way of thanking those people more warmly for their contribution.

Last and by no means least I wish to thank my family for generously allowing me time away from domestic duties to pen theses pages. I wish especially to thank Jane, my wife.

Part I

Setting Up the Replication Project

CHAPTER ONE

Recipe and Ingredients

Introduction

It is May 1997, and we are in the Department of Health again. It is almost exactly a year after the idea of 'Hendersons' in the North, South, East and West was conceived there. Then, we had been told that national funding could be available only if the new and expanded Henderson Hospital service for severe personality disorder (PD) covers all four corners of the country. It is surprising therefore that the Department of Health is now asking us to consider setting up just one other service. Also, the current proposal is that Henderson itself would not be centrally funded. We decline this new, less than generous, offer, making it clear that the whole deal is off if there are fewer than two new services and if Henderson is not also nationally funded. We argue that the independent research (to validate or otherwise the success of the replication process) would be compromised were there to be just Henderson and one other. There would be fewer lessons to be learnt from the setting up of a single new service, rather than two or more. Evaluating at least two new services in relation to Henderson, we contend, would confer advantage and could contribute evidence about service development that might be generaliseable elsewhere in the NHS.

On 23 October 1997, nearly a year after the original bid to the Department of Health (DH) was submitted, the deal is back on, though modified. We hear that central funding by the National Specialist Commissioning Advisory Group (NSCAG) has been granted for Henderson plus two new services. Joining us in St Helier NHS Trust are our partners from South Birmingham Mental Health NHS Trust and Mental Health Services of Salford NHS Trust (MHSS). The Department of Health's press release heralds: '£12M BOOST BRINGS NEW TREAT-MENTS TO NHS CENTRES OF EXCELLENCE'.

But, then, NSCAG requests that we delay the start, to enable government money actually to become available. (Only a portion of this £12 million was destined for the PD services at this point.) Frustrated, but secretly relieved, we indicate that we can accommodate their request. This hiatus gives us more time to plan, and we start a search for models of services that have successfully propagated. It also affords time for the reality of the situation to start to sink in.

The recipe book

TC literature

We hoped that the TC literature would help us with defining our replication task, indicating the steps by which to proceed. Much had been written about the 'experiments' carried out at Northfield and Mill Hill, where the prototype TCs were developed during, and after, World War II (Harrison and Clark 1992). This literature makes for absorbing reading for both the TC enthusiast and medical historian. Indeed, a special edition of *Therapeutic Communities: The International Journal for Therapeutic and Supportive Organisations* was devoted to the contributions of these pioneers (Kennard 1996). This literature describes the exhilaration of being at the forefront of a social movement, which questioned the prevailing assumptions about mental illness and treatment. Looking back over his 37 years involvement with TCs, Maxwell Jones describes how:

> ...the most important lesson of my life was the twelve years [1947–59] spent with 'sociopaths' at Belmont Hospital, later renamed Henderson Hospital, near London. We knew of no effective 'treatment' for this condition and had to turn to the 'patients' for help. Thus started the chain reaction of daily community meetings with all 'patients' and staff present (approximately 100 people), information-sharing, identification of problems, setting priorities, and shared decision-making, if possible reaching consensus...this experiment was forced on us by the very fact of our ignorance, but might one not extrapolate and suggest that all 'treatment' units might follow this pattern and attempt a fresh start, questioning all their preconceptions and prejudices, and involving the 'patients' as people from the start...? (Jones 1979, p. 34)

Reading such stirring stuff, sadly, did not help much. Not only were we not finding the recipe book. We were becoming increasingly worried that we did not know where the kitchen was! There is a difference between being at the start of the TC 'movement' (as were Maxwell Jones and his contemporaries) and being at the start of a project to replicate what had, in effect, become a routinised treatment approach (Manning 1989). In his book *The Therapeutic Community Movement: Charisma and Routinization*, Manning identifies a 'tension' that exists between 'innovation and routine'. Accordingly, what confronted our partnership bent on replication was this: How could we innovate (set up something where there had been nothing) and yet base this on something established, i.e. 'old' Henderson? Those involved in the project would need an inspiring, charismatic leaders – a Maxwell Jones or a Tom Main, but also the bureaucratic savvy to construct this new creation within the constraints posed by the modern, increasingly risk-averse NHS.

Setting up new TCs required us to be aware of the ideological underpinnings of such unusual healthcare organisations, the influence of this cultural heritage on the organisational structures and the way in which the blending of culture and structure could be understood in relation to the PD clients treated.

Ideology and history

During World War II it had become clear that the high level of healthcare demands posed by the vast number of psychological casualties among military personnel greatly outstripped the supply of relevant psychiatric services. (The modern range of psychotropic drugs had not yet been invented. Leaving aside ECT (electro-convulsive therapy), modified narcosis and insulin coma therapies, the main treatments were the so-called psychological or 'talking' treatments.) Being highly labour-intensive, existing psychological treatment could not contribute much to the supply side. New therapeutic inventions were required. Although they were founded on differing ideologies they had many aspects in common. In essence they were 'group' therapies. At a stroke, they yielded an improved staff:patient ratio. There was an enhanced capacity to treat the thousands of (non-psychotic) service personnel who had been shepherded into various military hospitals.

The 'experiments' taking place at Northfield Military Hospital in Birmingham are well described and derive from the collective talents of many who would distinguish themselves subsequently in their fields – Rickman, Bion, Foulkes, Bridger and Main – to name but the most famous. Between them they established the foundations of group psychotherapy (mainly under the leadership of Major Foulkes) and the therapeutic community, a term coined by Lt.-Colonel Main but a development credited to a range of individuals working around the same time, especially Maxwell Jones (Main 1983). The latter's approach (first in Dartford, then at Mill Hill) was to teach those patients who wrongly believed they had cardiac pathology on the basis of their symptoms (pain on exertion, shortness of breath, etc.) an understanding of rudimentary anatomy and physiology. They might then appreciate better how the cause of their symptoms was not cardiac in origin, hence not literally life-threatening (Jones 1952).

Jones's simple but seminal observation was that those 'students' (patients) in his classes who had been there longest could educate their neophyte fellows better than could the professionals, including himself, alone. This apparently mundane finding was to become for him the cornerstone of a democratic TC approach that put patients centre stage. In his hands it would lead to a radical overhaul of the traditional mental hospital's hierarchical relationships both between different staff disciplines and also between staff and patients. In taking on those patients for whom others had little to offer, he sowed the seeds for the later TC developments in the field of personality disorder. After the war, Jones moved to Belmont Hospital in Surrey (the site of the current Henderson Hospital) and put into practice what he had learnt at Mill Hill and even before that at Dartford (see Briggs 2003).

The unit that Jones established was funded as an experiment by the then Ministry of Labour, in collaboration with the Ministry of Health, to treat active service people having difficulty returning to 'Civvy Street'. Many of them had not enjoyed a place in society even before the war. These patients have been variously described and categorised (see Whiteley 1980). There was argument about whether the treatment was successful, as Jones claimed, and, if so, whether it was 'the man or the method' that was responsible. Early results of service evaluation, though encouraging, had been derived from clinical impressions and no comparison groups had been studied. Although some hard data regarding employment status were reported, in the absence of adequate controlled populations, no firm conclusions could be drawn (Jones 1952).

A culture of enquiry

Tom Main had indicated that it was the 'culture' rather than the 'structure' of the TC that formed its defining ingredient (Main 1983). However, as with the 'genes versus environment' debate, it is not really an either/or. Neither culture nor structure can exist in isolation. They are interactively present together and can only ever be artificially separated (Norton 1992). In setting out to replicate a TC, we concluded that it was the culture – a certain set of aims and values – that should determine the emergent structure (Manning and Blake 1979). The developing structure serves to influence the culture, and an iterative cycle is established. As Manning and Blake point out, there is then a challenge to the TC 'to maintain a clear view as to overall objectives, so that constructive change may be separated from that which is destructive' (p.157). For us there remained the twin issues of how best to introduce the required cultural elements and how these might induce a suitable structure that would feed back constructively on the unit's culture and still be recognisably 'Henderson'.

Although the culture of a TC is more or less straightforward to define – it relates to atmosphere, values held and embodied – infusing a new staff team and new institution with it and monitoring its emerging presence is problematic. It is far easier to instigate and measure structural forms, such as the presence and frequency of community meetings or communal meals. Yet the TC literature seems clear, agreeing with Tom Main, that it is the 'culture' rather than the 'structure' of an institution purporting to be a TC that is decisive. For Main, a TC represents a 'culture of enquiry...into personal and interpersonal and inter-system problems and a study of impulses, defences and relations as these are expressed and arranged socially' (Main 1983, p.217). This culture is easily lost, deteriorating into mindless rote memorising or becoming too inward looking (see Roberts 1980), and not so easy to re-instate once lost. The cut and thrust of the clinical day reveals this fragility and difficulty, although there is not necessarily ready agreement about its presence or absence at a given point in time (Norton 1992). In setting up new TCs we needed a reference point, and there seemed none better than to consider what values and ideologies the Rapoport team had found at Henderson when they studied it in the late 1950s. This might be as close as we could get to finding a recipe. It might help us to identify ingredients needed for the 'sauce', if falling short of supplying the 'meat' or providing the necessary cooking utensils and instructions.

Henderson's cultural heritage

Rapoport's team of social anthropologists studied the TC developed at Henderson Hospital over a period of years. Theirs was an in-depth study of its method, even though their original brief had been to evaluate outcome (Whiteley 1980). The study is particularly remembered for its delineation, using an interview and questionnaire method, of a set of ideologies that typified the staff then working at the Unit – permissiveness, democratisation, communalism and reality confrontation (Rapoport 1960). These terms are not always understood fully, nor is it always appreciated that these ideological positions, in practice, do not readily harmonise. For example, there can be a tension between permissiveness (meaning a tendency towards greater tolerance within the TC than is found in the wider society outside of hospital) and reality confrontation. The latter requires the individual to be presented with the honest feedback of others, especially in relation to the negative effects of their frequently anti-social or asocial attitudes or actions.

'Democratisation' stands for the delegation of some important aspects of the staff's traditional authority, responsibility and decision-making power to the client group. An example of this at Henderson is the joint involvement of patients and staff in both the selection and discharge from hospital of fellow patients, with patients having the larger say by virtue of their greater number, hence higher number of votes to cast. While staff may have no difficulty with democratisation as an idea, translating such theory into practice is not necessarily straightforward. If staff believe that a patient may be on the brink of discharge from treatment, due to what they perceive to be the effect of scapegoating by the patient group, it can be hard for them to remain committed to the ideal of the majority being always in the right. Also, the cosy rhetoric of 'communalism', the joint participation in tasks by staff and patients (such as the selection and discharge of clients, but also cleaning, gardening and maintenance of the building), may appear less attractive in practice than in theory. Most staff prefer to choose not only the clients with whom they work but also the nature of that work.

Nevertheless, it is clearly desirable that staff have ideals compatible with the carrying out of the therapeutic work in a democratic TC (Kennard 1989). In a paper entitled 'Towards a theory for milieu treatment of hospitalised borderline patients', Svein Haugsgjerd (a Norwegian psychotherapist) identifies the central importance of a shared philosophy. The latter is represented by 'fundamental ideas' that he subsumes under five headings: (1) the importance of the staff group as a unified work group; (2) a shared epistemological orientation; (3) shared ideas about mental health as being trust in verbal communication and ability to keep divergent ideas and emotions in the mind without splitting and projection all the time; (4) some basic Kleinian and Bionian concepts about psychopathology, the self-curative tendency, and the therapeutic process; (5) emphasis on an actual understanding (and not-understanding), excepting that our understanding is limited and in constant flux (Hargsgjerd 1987).

When I started out on the 1997 TC development project, I did not know this work. However, its 'fundamental ideas' are in accord with those embodied at Henderson. To a degree, these ideas complement the four ideological themes described by Rapoport and colleagues and stand for a partial unpacking of them. Kennard's 'democratic tendency', a term he borrows from Winnicott, also captures something of the essence of the Henderson staff team's shared ideology (Kennard 1989). Such writings gave us cause for optimism that it might also prove possible to identify individuals having this personality attribute. If so, such staff members should be able to contribute to a multi-disciplinary team in which the traditional hierarchical structure, particularly between staff and clients, was to be flattened (Jones 1952).

Structure and culture in relation to clientele

We believed that we would need to convey to the staff in the new services not only the 'what to do' but also the 'why to do it'. This was necessary since some were likely to be unfamiliar with the TC method of working in a deep collaboration with both colleagues and clients. However, at the start of this replication project we were not clear about the 'core' features of the model, those essential to replicate, and how these related to residents' psychopathology, individually and collectively. To an extent we are still in the dark, although the replication process itself has shed some valuable light on this relationship – between the structure of the therapeutic programme and the psychopathology of the clientele. What follows is my attempt to describe the 'structure' of the Henderson's democratic TC and its relevance to a personality disordered clientele.

From the mid-1960s, the emphasis at Henderson has been on providing treatment for people suffering from personality disorder. No psychotropic drugs are prescribed and all treatment is group-based. There is an intensive mix of group ingredients, including community meetings (six per week), small psycho-therapy groups (three per week), psychodrama (weekly), art therapy (weekly), work groups (twice weekly), 'welfare groups' (one or two times per week) and groups set up specifically to support joining and leaving the community (Table 1.1; and see Norton 1992b). As well as this formal programme of meetings there is an expectation that all members take on 'jobs', i.e. specific roles within the TC for its necessary functioning, for example the ordering, storing and cooking of the TC's food. Most of the posts have an assistant so that there is a graded entry into the TC according to seniority. This provides a gradual familiarisation with

Table 1.1 Weekly programme at the Henderson Hospital

WEEKLY PROGRAMME

MONDAY	TUESDAY	WEDNESDAY	THURSDAY	FRIDAY	SATURDAY	SUNDAY
9.15–10.30 a.m.		'9.15' COMMUNITY MEETING				
10.30 a.m.		MORNING BREAK				
Small groups New residents' group	Cleaning and reviews or elections or community projects	Small groups New residents' group Leavers' transition group	Visitors' group* Women's group Men's group	Small groups New residents' group		
11.00–12.00 noon	11.00–12.00 noon	10.30–11.30 a.m.	11.00–12.00 noon	11.00–12.00 noon		
12.15–12.30 p.m.		CLEANING				
12.30 p.m.		LUNCH BREAK				
Surgery 1.00–1.30 p.m.	Surgery 2.05–2.15 p.m.	Surgery 2.05–2.15 p.m.	Surgery 2.05–2.15 p.m.	Surgery 2.05–2.15 p.m.	Weekdays Welfare phone slot 10.30 a.m.–11.00 a.m. 12.30 p.m.–1.00 p.m.	
Floor reps meeting 1.30–1.45 p.m. Sports and social 1.45–2.10 p.m. Research meeting 1.30–2.00 p.m.						

Continued on next page

Table 1.1 cont.

WEEKLY PROGRAMME

	MONDAY	TUESDAY	WEDNESDAY	THURSDAY	FRIDAY	SATURDAY	SUNDAY
	Psychodrama or art therapy	Selection/unit reception or welfare or sports and social	Psychodrama or art therapy	Work groups (art, welfare or gardening and maintenance)	Work groups (art, welfare or gardening and maintenance)		
	2.30–4.15 p.m.	2.30–4.15 p.m.	2.30–4.15 p.m.	2.15–4.15 p.m.	2.15–4.15 p.m.		
					Tea 4.30–5.00 p.m.		
5.00 p.m.	HANDOVER						
7.00–9.00 p.m.	COMMUNITY MEAL						
9.45–10.30 p.m.	SUMMIT MEETING (Top 4 residents and staff)						9.45–10.30 p.m. Summit
							10.05 p.m. Booking in
11.00 p.m.	NIGHT ROUND						

* Visitors' Day (Professional visitors) – Thursday 8.45 a.m.–5.00 p.m. Community Afternoon – last Thursday in month 2.15–4.15 p.m.

the tasks required to service the TC. Individuals can nominate themselves for the roles or be nominated but it is only the peer group that can vote to indicate if there is sufficient 'confidence' in the nominee to fulfil the position. Crucially, the tasks are carried out with others rather than in a solitary fashion, thereby necessitating 'interaction' (see later and Whiteley 1986).

The informal time between group meetings is integral to the treatment rather than separate from or just an adjunct to it (see Hinshelwood 1988 for a discussion of this topic). Research has also borne out this belief at least to an extent (Whiteley and Collis 1987). It was found that clients located the most important therapeutic 'events' as being more often during the informal time than in the formal programme. This might partially reflect the fact that an emergency meeting of the whole TC can be called at any time of the day or night, but is usually during informal time. This 'referred meeting' takes precedence over any other activity and requires all who have been notified of it – 'referred' – to attend. Clients risk being discharged if they fail to attend. The close temporal proximity of such a meeting to the issue or event provoking it – usually some major upset or episode of destructive behaviour – means an enhanced learning potential from the experience, as compared to other types of (non-TC) psychiatric or penal settings.

The TC environment thus yields an experience of 'living-learning' (Maxwell Jones's term) facilitated, in part, via the community's judicious calling of emergency meetings of and for itself. These often serve to underline the importance of events occurring between the group meetings of the formal programme. This process models a mature reflection on events and situations and allows for judgements about priorities to be made – both qualities that are often lacking in clients embarking on therapy. A cycle of 'interacting', 'exploring' motivations, especially via the peer group, and 'experimenting' with new ways of coping (especially during the social time) characterises the therapeutic process (Whiteley 1986). Staff are involved both in the formal programme and during 'social' time, but the idea is that they avoid taking on a direct leadership function in most situations.

The Henderson staff team is multi-disciplinary and relates to its four major functions – clinical work of the residential TC; preparation and aftercare (outreach function); staff consultation, education and supervision (training function); and evaluation (audit and research function). Staffing a 24 hours per day, seven days per week, residential unit is resource-intensive. However, at night (from 5 p.m. to 9 a.m.) the staff is pared down to a minimum, with just two members on duty – usually one senior Charge Nurse and one Social Therapist (see below). Such staff comprise the 'rota staff', as compared to those simply working '9 to 5', Monday to Friday. Seventy-six per cent of the week is non-9 to 5, so, for the vast majority of time, it is the resident groups (up to 29 resident members) who comprise the community and regulate its clinical function. (Senior '9 to 5' staff are available on-call for advice at all times.)

New staff enjoy an extended induction through attending specifically designed weekly training and supervision sessions convened by senior Henderson personnel. This supports the apprenticeship model that schools new staff members into the TC's unusual therapeutic methods. All clinical work takes place in group settings, and each of these is facilitated by a multi-disciplinary group of staff, usually three in number. This provides the necessary continuity of staffing and protects individual staff members from over-exposure to the client group, whose interaction can be stressful (Miller 1989).

The two night staff hand over relevant information from their 16-hour shift to the incoming '9 to 5' and rota staff – the latter usually work a single night shift per week, with the rest of their hours being made up of Monday to Friday (plus occasional weekend shifts). Thus the whole multi-disciplinary staff team on duty on a given weekday – approximately ten in number – meet as a team to receive the 'handover' from 8.50 a.m. to 9.10 a.m. This can be a time-pressured encounter, depending upon what and how much has happened during the night shift. Its purpose is to maintain continuity of approach, to ensure adequate inter-staff communication about relevant issues – especially in relation to 'risk' – and to prepare staff for what to expect of the residents on a given day.

For staff, the working day of the clinical timetable (Table 1.1) is interspersed with staff meetings, including so-called 'after-groups'. The latter follow all clinical meetings and allow participating staff to ventilate feelings, attempt to understand the clinical material and offer peer support and supervision to one another, as required. Ideally there is a spread of seniority and discipline among the staffing of any particular group component. The whole clinical staff team meets after all community meetings, emergency meetings and at each lunchtime – the latter meetings last for one hour. Two of such staff meetings – 'supervision' and 'team awareness' – happen with external facilitation, through a suitably qualified professional who works outside of Henderson, indeed outside of our NHS Trust.

The externally facilitated groups are central to keeping alive the 'culture of enquiry' referred to above. The fact of their being facilitated by non-Henderson individuals (not the same person for supervision as for team awareness) helps the staff team avoid being too inward-looking or preoccupied with TC method or details. These structures diminish the likelihood of missing the 'bigger picture' or, on the other hand, being inattentive or over-attentive to particular issues or individual residents. The nature of the day-to-day work, the inter-connectedness of structure and culture, might emerge more clearly in the ensuing sections of this chapter.

As described above, much was known about the structure of the current Henderson – the composition of its staff team, the therapeutic programme, the 'jobs' undertaken by patients, the integration of the informal time and the precedence taken by the emergency meetings. However, what was less certain was (1) how these could be created in the new services so as to achieve a suitable 'culture' and (2) how the new staff could be taught, within the time available, to undertake the teamwork in a similar fashion to that of Henderson, taking into account both structural and cultural elements. Worryingly, for those of us tasked with replicating Henderson, it was not clear whether only some or all of the above structural ingredients were actually necessary. Nor was it clear how important it might be that managerial structures, not just clinical structures, were replicated. Jones had commented that to be successful TCs needed 'sanctions from above…[as well as] psycho-dynamic skills, commitment, and courage to face the inevitable resistance to change'. This is because 'to develop such an open system [as that of the TC] strikes at the very roots of our culture' (Jones 1952, p.9). Only time would tell.

We knew that the required 'culture of enquiry' could not reside exclusively in any solitary staff member, no matter how inclined towards democracy and dedicated to the flattening of hierarchies or blurring of staff roles within the multi-disciplinary staff team. It would not even be the sole prerogative of the staff team, even if working together successfully to facilitate particular 'groups' within the overall programme. It would be the result of a combination of many influences, in particular the interaction between the staff and resident 'sub-systems'. Therefore, the challenge was to create both a formal structured group programme (and interleafed informal times – an integrated whole) that could become self-reflective and still be active and productive enough to perform its basic functions. This functioning interpersonal environment would need to imbibe and expel its resident members according to its rules. Residents would be admitted and discharged as directed by the TC. We were aiming to produce 'community as doctor', as Rapoport's team had so aptly named their publication concerning Henderson's therapeutic processes.

A replicated Henderson would need to scrutinise itself and, during the more painful periods of that undertaking, be sufficiently supported by the management structures, within and outside of itself, so to do. All of this was to be achieved, incidentally, at a time when the prevailing management culture was one of risk-aversion. The latter would be evidenced later by difficulties with, and reluctance about, replication in relation to: the staff shift pattern (for fear of contravening an EC directive, even though the Trust's legal department had given the go-ahead); inclusion criteria for referrals (in relation to age cut-offs and criminal offence history); and even the practice of patients ordering, storing and cooking food for the TC, without the involvement of staff to oversee the process at every stage.

For Henderson's structure to be absorbed, so that it might impact appropriately on the culture, it had to be rendered digestible. It is relatively easy to illustrate the treatment programme diagrammatically (see Table 1.1). Also, it has been advocated that, to an extent, each successive 24-hour period should be construed as a single therapeutic session, albeit a long one, since staff are required to hold in mind a transference-countertransference paradigm and to support this capacity in colleagues (Whiteley 1978). However, the absence of a theoretical model of personality disorder that could neatly unpack into the structural elements of the TC was a weakness – one which would be pointed out by the Director of one of the new services. Therefore, the new staff would need to learn, to an extent, by rote, what were the necessary TC structures. Only later, and slowly, might they understand the relevance of these structures to the overall, year-long treatment package and to the profound interpersonal inadequacy that is the trademark of severe PD (Holmes 1999).

The clients

Once admitted, Henderson's clients are referred to and known as 'residents', a term which denotes their status as those residing as opposed to merely working in the TC and which conveys the sense of a more active participation in their therapy than does the term 'patient'. The new services not only had new staff but a group of potential new residents who were, like the staff, being 'fast-tracked' in order to 'hit the ground running' on the very first day of the service opening. This client group, said not to learn from experience and not to be able to delay gratification, we expected to be able to collaborate with new staff, at least to an extent, in order for there to be any real chance of realising a functioning TC. Inevitably, there was a degree of mismatch between our expectation and their actual capacity, given the nature of this personality disordered client group (see Table 1.2 denoting aspects of past history as reported by referring professionals).

Table 1.2 Characteristics of consecutive admissions to Henderson Hospital (n=238)

Feature	Number	Per cent
Gender (Female)	127	53.4
Ethnicity (white)	225	94.5
Marital status (single)	186	78.2
Employed	25	10.5
Inpatient treatment (past)	148	62.2
Outpatient treatment (past)	169	71.0
Previous convictions	100	42.0
Suicide attempts	133	55.9
Overdoses	147	61.8
Self-mutilation	124	52.1
Alcohol abuse	124	52.1
Drug abuse	98	41.2

At Henderson, clients will have been resident for at least three months before taking on the more responsible roles within the programme. This will have allowed them both to experience the system and to witness others operating it, to greater or lesser effect. For their term of office they thus enter the situation relatively well prepared, even though there is no substitute for the experience of doing the most senior jobs, such as the 'Top Three' (this term denotes the three senior residents elected to occupy the most influential of residents' jobs that include chairing the community meetings, chairing the selection groups and convening and chairing the emergency meetings that deal with crises – see below). This situation would not and could not be the case with the new services.

A central TC notion is the enactment of ordinary everyday life but inside the institution of the TC – the reproduction of 'social reality' (Main 1946). Via this route the clients' interpersonal problems can be encountered and understood. Paradoxically, clients are 'required' to enact their problems and not to avoid them or leave them behind in the outside world. This approach would not be necessary had they a capacity to present their difficulties verbally and with appropriate feeling. Neither of these capacities being firmly established – thoughts and feelings are often dislocated from one another – necessitates a different therapeutic stance from that of traditional psychiatry. Being selected for admission, and accepting this offer, amounts to the future resident's acceptance of an informal (and unwritten) contract to attempt genuinely to live by the community's rules – a microcosm of those of the wider society – and to participate in the social life, as well as the formal treatment programme, of the TC. These contractual requirements pose a fundamental problem for PD clients. In so doing, a positive expectation is imparted – they have some capacity for healthy psychosocial functioning. Therefore living in the TC, for up to one year, represents a therapeutic opportunity as well as challenge. There is no expectation that new clients know how the TC functions or will be able simply to abide by the rules and participate. Rather there is an expectation that the more senior residents will actively inform and support new arrivals to acclimatise and settle – as originally observed by Maxwell Jones in Dartford and applied at Mill Hill and Henderson. In so doing they may imbibe the democratic and 'social' ways of Henderson, hence of wider society.

The whole and the sum of its parts

The TC can be construed as a single holistic entity. However, the notion of wholeness is more an ideal to be striven for than an achievable everyday reality (Norton 2003). In as much as the TC fails to operate in an integrated manner, its therapeutic potential remains unfulfilled. Paradoxically, the client group functions often as if to render the TC merely an assortment of disconnected and meaningless fragments, reminiscent of the residents' formative experiences during childhood, often repeated long into adulthood. It is also possible for staff, largely unwittingly, to contribute to processes that are destructive to the overall therapeutic functioning of the TC. These matters will be discussed in detail later (Chapter 3). At this juncture, however, it is relevant to consider how the residents' psycho-pathology (especially in its interpersonal manifestation) has its TC structural counterpart, designed to provide short-term safe containment and longer-term insight. Although this correspondence of psychopathology with structure is far from exact, considering it from such a perspective can provide the reader with something of a rationale for the way things are organised within the democratic TC that is the Henderson.

Identity diffusion meets reality confrontation

Erikson (Erikson 1956) referred to individuals who are incapacitated by not knowing how they stand in relation to others with whom they come into contact or, as importantly, how they stand in relation to themselves. Their internal worlds tend to be marked by extremes. They may oscillate thus between feeling wound up in a 'whirlwind' or else becalmed – 'down in the doldrums' (Norton 1997a). What evokes or provokes such extreme states or why one extreme rather than the other holds sway is seldom understood. Such individuals tend to feel as if swept along in a disorienting intra-psychic and interpersonal world, wherein little of stability and meaning is apprehended, from which rescue is sought.

Individuals with severe PD have a poorly integrated concept of self and of significant others (Kernberg 1986). Often abruptly and uncomfortably, they move from one extreme view of themselves and others to the opposite pole, sometimes with little or no time between – moving from pillar to post. Not only are others unable to understand fully the mental contortions but the 'subject' is also often confused. It is little surprise therefore that the PD individual seeks extreme solutions to provide some respite from such a stormy internal world. These are usually aggressive and destructive strategies or else passive-aggressive ones, including with the 'self' as victim. Professionals involved may feel drawn into the drama or pulled out of their usual role, only to be left ultimately paralysed and defeated in pursuit of a therapeutic outcome.

The trademark of Henderson's democratic TC is its ability to make the total community resource available at short notice, via an emergency (referred) meeting, at any time of day or night. In this it is unmatched by traditional psychi-atric wards or units. The speed of its response, coupled with the range and com-plexity of support and challenge delivered as 'feedback' during it (reality con-frontation), especially from the peer group, makes this a powerful intervention in relation to the clients' sense of self and others. The fact that the response is quick sends the residents a clear message that they exist, since their behaviour is clearly shown to impact on others. The fact that the message from those on the receiving end is clear and direct, as well as complex – it represents a mix of support and challenge – provides the individual with food for thought. The latter would be less digestible were the feedback to derive merely from professionals. The client's peer group is potentially influential and the public nature of the group-work forum affords opportunities for others to learn vicariously about themselves and others.

Feedback from the resident's peer group can be delivered in an authentic and genuine manner, not always available to staff. Its clinical significance derives from the fact of it coming from people who are (relatively) trusted, respected and valued and whose positive regard is therefore desired. The immediacy and strength of feeling often enacted, particularly in the emergency meeting, differs in its directness from the usual institutional contact with professionals. The latter can become hardened and apparently or actually unresponsive. Alternatively they may be over-solicitous in order to avoid showing any negativity. Such extreme and partial responses themselves may result in the client not feeling genuinely understood – as a whole – and can provoke an escalation of the client's destructive and provocative behaviour, in seeking to obtain a more authentic response from staff. Literally vicious cycles can ensue.

Discontinuity of experience meets integration of groups

We all tend to cling to what we know. Often this involves ignoring contrary evidence and the opinions of others, including so-called experts. This tendency is especially prevalent amongst Henderson's PD clients. The reason for this probably stems from their basic mistrust of others, as well as an impaired tolerance of anxiety that would be engendered were new evidence, conflicting with past 'wisdom', to be entertained seriously. PD individuals do not tend to experience themselves as embedded in a secure 'present', which derives from an understandable past, and from which an expectable future can be contemplated (Lambert 1981). In the face of 'conflicting' new evidence, the usual defences are erected and anxiety avoided, albeit at the expense of learning. The result is that existing beliefs and attitudes persist unchanged. The fact of this personality predisposition poses a challenge for the TC and so there are structures set up to counter it.

The particular structural solutions to this personality predisposition, however, are deceptively simple. They include the nightly meeting of the four senior elected residents whose job it is to review the events of the day with the two duty staff who are working the night shift, and three standing items on the morning community meeting – emergency meeting feedback, 'summit' meeting feedback and feedback from small groups attended the previous day. Yet what these structural ingredients represent poses a challenge to the residents, since it requires them to think about what went on in the past – as recently as yesterday – and to think about themselves and others in relation to it. It will come as no surprise to the reader that the smooth and effective functioning of these particular structures is problematic. Departures and deviations from the advertised structure (see Table 1.3) abound.

Table 1.3 Community meeting agenda

Item	Matters concerning
'Good morning'	
Who's missing?	Resident (or assistant) to report absentees
Handover (rota'd clients)	Residents to take part in 5 p.m. handover to staff
Wash-ups (rota'd clients)	Lunch, tea, supper (daily)
Supper – vegetarian – meat	Cooks – volunteers, not involved in wash-ups
Staff feedback	Staff absence (leave, sickness, etc.), other staff movements, issues not otherwise covered on agenda
'Referred' and yesterday's feedback	Emergency meetings, and unstructured time fed back
Groups' feedback	Previous day's groups fed back
Summit discussed	Summit meeting topics fed back to rest of community
Groups, votes, and why?	Report on those who missed groups or broke major rules
Ask for sleeping-in extensions	Those technically discharged by rule-breaking seek temporary re-instatement
Votes taken	Democratic votes to ascertain whether a resident is discharged for rule-breaking
Emergency extensions	Asking community's permission to miss group activity
Meeting closed	

Frequently, the time set aside at the 'summit' meeting, to review the events of the previous day, is used for other purposes: arguing about an apparently trivial disagreement between the two staff and the four residents; avoiding the main and obvious item to be discussed, perhaps discussing another topic to its exclusion – filibustering – and arranging for an emergency meeting to intrude on the time available or at least doing nothing to avoid this outcome. At the next day's community meeting, when the discussion from summit is fed back, there are still things that can stand in the way of a linkage between thoughts and feelings. For example, even though the emergency meetings are all 'minuted', they may be read out to the community in such a way as to render them meaningless and difficult to attend to. Alternatively, the account of events may be so detailed, or the rendition so slow, that insufficient time is left, in a tightly packed agenda, to do justice to the matters in hand. If the meeting is faithfully reported and re-presented, there are still many avoidant directions that can be taken that are more or less subtle. Blaming staff, for example, for inappropriately suggesting that the matter is discussed at all, is a favourite. But there are many more: an argument over some concrete detail may be embellished and used to take up the time; the facts of the matter may be disagreed – either between two protagonists or involving many or most of the resident sub-system of the community; a person involved may be challenged about another matter altogether; friends of those involved may take up the matter, sidelining those actually involved, etc., etc. Some of these manoeuvrings are no doubt quite conscious, but others appear to be less so. However, staff are taxed to tell the difference and to find ways of getting an issue or individual addressed so as to allow mature reflection – to achieve genuine linkage.

With the 'summit discussed' item, the person introducing the headlines of the discussion may not have been actually present. The scene may then be set, not for a discussion but a rapidly degenerating row, in which the current community meeting is distracted from the issues concerned. Alternatively, as is often the case, the summary may be delivered so cryptically that only those expert at crosswords stand any chance of deciphering what had actually gone on in the meeting the night before. Sometimes the chairperson is left with no support from the fellow residents who had been present the previous night, in addressing what might be a sensitive issue. An example might be telling a member of the community that his or her hygiene leaves something to be desired. Of course, if the earlier summit meeting itself ran into problems, of whatever kind, then it is more likely that something untoward will occur in the relaying of the content of that meeting in the following day's community meeting. The smaller therapy groups are not recorded in writing and what is fed back will depend on the group memory, notoriously unreliable and subject to distortion.

Many of the above examples are commonplace and may appear unremarkable. This they are. Yet they are also the very stuff of everyday relationships – representative of the reasons that brought the residents into the TC in the first place. What the TC offers therefore is something that is relevant but significantly different from what has been experienced before. There will be opportunities for those whose voice was never listened to previously to find that they can get a hearing – especially if they have demonstrated some commitment to the TC by virtue of taking on elected jobs or contributing in other ways to the informal life of the TC. Those used to an environment in which only those who speak loudest get heard will find that the norm is different at Henderson with bullying or hectoring challenged and going largely unrewarded. Sometimes it is left to the staff to ensure that no two people talk at the same time, pointing out the obvious difficulty in hearing the important words that each may be saying. Anger is so much easier for many of the residents to express than is sadness or a simple request for support – often experienced as intensely humiliating. It is the linking of such emotions as depression, fear, humiliation and shame to events – recent or remote – that is so difficult and so readily avoided both consciously and unconsciously.

Impulsivity meets planned action and play

The majority of Henderson's TC 24-hour day is unstructured. To most residents, even those who protest that they have to attend so many therapy groups, this is a difficult time. Residents are relatively poor at entertaining or even occupying themselves in the absence of ready-made entertainment, such as a TV soap on the communal set, an emergency meeting or some other real-life drama played out in the TC. Residents are also poor at 'self-soothing'. In the past they readily turned for relief to substances, such as illicit or prescribed drugs, or to actions, such as violence against the self or others. It is especially, therefore, between groups in the informal time that residents experience an urge to resort to their usual coping strategies. For many, on account of past trauma, nighttime is the worst time. It is, of course, relatively easy to disguise this (often shameful) secret from others. However, with time, at least the more gross difficulties with sleeping tend to be uncovered or disclosed – an advantage of the residential situation over partial hospitalisation or outpatient alternatives.

In order to help residents deal with their impulses there is a range of structures: sports facilities and a once-weekly group to facilitate interactive activity of a sporting or other game-playing kind; work groups that also rely to an extent on the expenditure of physical energy and activity, allowing a positive outlet for normal impulses to action; art therapy and psychodrama, both of which provide for the expression of impulses via non-verbal means. These may help clients to communicate something of their internal state not otherwise easily communicable in words. In the weekly psychodrama session it may be possible to experiment actively with 'alternative' pasts, presents and futures, in the service of trying to understand the personal and interpersonal implications via concrete enactment.

Many of Henderson's clients inhabit a timeless world dominated by impulses and unrealistic expectations of others, who as a result are seen erroneously to be in a position to respond creatively to the clients' urgings. Omnipotent or else impotent fantasies, both conscious and unconscious, abound. The lack of suitable channels for pent-up energies means that, in the absence of their usual methods of coping, clients are often in a highly charged mental state, longing to discharge what is felt as excess energy or aching boredom. In the absence of sufficient prior experiences of containment of frustration and anger, there is a much diminished capacity for 'play' (Winnicott 1972, p.35). According to Winnicott, some individuals are unable to 'get excited while playing, and to feel satisfied with the game, without feeling threatened by a physical orgasm of local excitement'. Instead, 'the body becomes physically involved'. Uncontrollable urges are thus triggered in the course of even mundane daily activities. In the absence of an adequate capacity for sustained enjoyment, the game is no longer just a game. Mutual respect and fun are thus sacrificed on the altar of domination and power or alternatively submission and powerlessness – a passive-aggressive resolution of the problem.

Abandonment fears meet preparation for leaving

Most of Henderson's clients have experienced unsatisfactory separation and may have little or no experience of its satisfactory processing. They will have been seldom prepared for or desirous of the separation. Sometimes it will have arisen through family break-up and the intervention of social services, resulting in their removal to an institution or substitute family. It might have been enacted via expulsion from school or frequent moves, which both undermine education and fracture friendships. Untimely and sudden deaths also play a part. All leave ugly psychological scars that impress on a future that is consequently marked by a terror of proximity, of abandonment or, frequently, of both. The cocktail of identity diffusion, attacks on linking, discontinuity of experience of self, impulsivity and terror of abandonment guarantees problems not only with engaging in a therapeutic programme but with leaving it.

There are a number of structures to support both the practical and emotional aspects of joining and leaving the TC's year-long programme of treatment. Crucially, Henderson's 'outreach' function provides a 'before and after' service, to address a range of relevant concerns. These originally came to light via the undertaking of an audit of ex-residents, their referrers and family doctors (Dolan and Norton 1998). All concurred that more should have been, and could be, done to smooth the transition into and out of the TC, including both practical and emotional aspects.

For Henderson's new residents there is a thrice-weekly group to attend during the first three weeks. As well as residential and outreach staff there is a resident who is already established in the TC – a kind of 'buddy' – attending as part of a rota of more senior residents. This resident spends one week in that setting before attending the leavers' group in the following week and then returning full-time to their usual thrice-weekly small group (see Table 1.1). In the 'new residents' group are discussed practical issues to do with the TC's programme of therapy, the building, the rules and responsibilities and the systems of support that are available. In particular there is the need to foster understanding that the first port of call in the TC is usually another resident, not staff as with most of the other institutions with which the resident may have come into contact. Among residents it is especially the elected 'Top Three' who will begin to assume the position of authority figures in the new client's mind – not an easy transition for most. Many confess to difficulty leaving behind usual supports whether human (family, friends, etc.) or physical (drugs, alcohol, self-mutilation, etc.). Initially new residents are exempt from some of the manual tasks – cleaning, cooking and washing up – undertaken by the rest of the residents and do not have the 'vote' in their first week. Some welcome this as supportive, but others feel frustrated and excluded, all of which becomes the stuff of discussion in the new residents' group and elsewhere in and outside of groups.

Many clients have money worries (some serious debts), and there is often concern associated with social security benefits and the changes to them caused by coming into hospital. The senior residents are often the experts on such matters of state-derived funds. Their expertise is channelled formally through the twice-weekly 'welfare groups'. These meetings provide access to hospital tele-phones and to the advice of residents and staff, as well as providing support with difficult communication with outside authorities – technical and emotional diffi-culties. Groups are followed by an after-group, in which the residents can look at how it felt to do the business, whether support was asked for and, if it was, whether it helped. In this forum many are confronted with the stark reality of their difficulty with trusting others and their ingrained tendencies to go it alone, regardless of the ineffectiveness of such a strategy in the past.

Usually the welfare aspects are sorted with the support of the group and the residents will be able to start to settle, but it is often stressed that preparation for leaving the TC should begin almost from the outset. This is because many do not have stable or appropriate accommodation and do have significant financial problems. Few avail themselves of this advice, resulting in matters being left till prompted by the relevant structure, that of the 'leavers' group'. Residents are eligible to join this group three months prior to leaving. Some need encourage-ment to join it, and some only do so kicking and screaming, as it were!

A most helpful development in recent years has been the evolution of this group into the 'transition group'. The birth of this new group was not uncompli-cated but its incorporation of ex-residents – those in their first six months of freedom following their completed stay in the TC – has meant that thinking about the difficult reality of life after Henderson cannot easily be denied or postponed. Those who are due to leave hear of the life beyond and are helped thereby to make realistic plans for their future anticipated needs. Often, this is un-familiar emotional and intellectual territory. Noteworthy is the tendency for residents to divorce emotional from practical matters. Linking these is the work of the after-groups and community meetings into which information from the leavers' groups is fed (see 'Discontinuity of experience meets integration of groups' above).

Conclusions

The TC literature provided rich fare in its own way. However, deriving from different eras and starting points, it revealed little of direct relevance. There was no single or simple recipe to follow. The early TC origins were true innovations founded around charismatic individuals sharing important ideological aspects. The latter informed the emergent TC culture, inducting sympathetic structures via an interactive process. The particular challenge posed by the Henderson replication project was how to inject an ideology and culture into a newly appointed staff team, within a defined, relatively brief, period of time. The dependence of the Henderson model on the delegation of power and authority to the client group also created a difficulty. Not only would the individuals involved need to cohere as a unique team but they would also need to support the development of a similar ideology and culture in their clients.

We imagined that teaching new staff about the standard ingredients – the monthly timetable, the rules; the jobs; the formal hierarchy of residents (with 'Top Three' at the top of the pile) – would be relatively straightforward. It was the inculcation of the cultural aspects, however, which was our major concern. Ideally we would select staff who already had democratic tendencies. But these staff would need to maintain such a stance in the face of clinical pressures, emanating from their interaction with residents, which could wrest them from their professional roles and usual composure. The new staff would need to be team players, as it were, in two matches, more or less simultaneously – that of the staff team and of the whole TC, i.e. the mix of staff and residents. Those operating the 'rota', working at nights and weekends, as well as during the 9 to 5 programme, would genuinely need to embody such team spirit. It would therefore be crucial for new staff to gain an understanding of how the psychotherapy and sociotherapy aspects articulated with one another and how the structural–cultural blending (bearing the refining input of generations of residents) contained, confronted and supported residents in difficulties.

Those of us from Henderson embarking on the replication project were part of an existing whole creation – a kind of TC cake, if you like. However we had not been present at its conception or delivery. We certainly were not part of its original ingredients. We did not therefore understand how such ingredients had been identified and blended. Records were either absent or incomplete. Where present they reflected contexts which no longer existed. We remained acutely aware of the richness and complexity of our TC confection but under-confident of our ability to divine either the required ingredients or how to combine them under the conditions and constraints of the modern NHS 'kitchen'.

CHAPTER TWO

The Blending

Introduction

We had thought, in June 1998, that we had a relatively clear sense of the main structural and cultural ingredients that might inform a training curriculum. However, we had less idea about how to make these ingredients palatable to staff in the new settings – to design educational processes that would influence trainees so that they could imbibe such 'food for thought'. Therefore we – the Henderson Development Team (HDT) – decided to ask for outside expert help with the training task. Our chosen expert was Dr Brian Jolly, a medical educationalist, at the time based in Sheffield (now Professor, in Australia). He confirmed that we had indeed embarked upon an ambitious programme. Fortunately for us, this conclusion served to secure his enthusiastic support for our project.

Without an existing recipe and being ignorant of how to proceed, we had to start somewhere. We were a multi-disciplinary team of Project Manager, two Charge Nurses, two Social Therapists and myself. So, Rapoport's ideological statements – permissiveness, democratisation, communalism and reality confrontation (see p.21) seemed a logical starting point. However, it soon became clear that these 'themes' would need to be processed, so that they could be made digestible for teaching purposes. In a sense, we would be reversing the process that generated such thematic distillations. Rapoport's team of social anthropologists studying Henderson (over a period of years) had observed a range of 'behaviours', deducing from these what ideas/ideals lay behind them. We now were attempting to define behaviours that would reflect those same ideological themes and values. This would help develop our capacity to gather evidence (via observable 'behaviours' rated as present or absent) that the new staff had acquired relevant TC skills or not. To achieve this end we ourselves needed to be schooled in how to convert the ideology into rateable items and were duly disciplined by Jennie Harwood (a training consultant) in whose (firm) hands the aptly named Dr Jolly had placed us.

Initially and repeatedly, we failed to discriminate adequately the 'whats' of the potential curriculum from the 'hows' of its delivery. Jennie (a competent horsewoman and taker of exotic and dangerous holidays) spurred us into unfamiliar intellectual territory. In the process we were not allowed to be reflectively vague or free associative, as was our psychotherapeutic penchant. We had to break down the four ideological themes of Rapoport into discrete and identifiable knowledge, attitudes and behaviours. We had to be crystal clear about the 'what' that we wanted the new trainees to learn. Time and again, we would stray into describing 'how' we might achieve the 'what', only to find ourselves sharply whipped into line by the horsewoman. Mostly we took such chiding in good part, but it was clear that Jennie was determined and that, although we were paying her, she called the shots – rather repetitive ones: 'That's a "how" not a "what"!' It was kind of fun, some of the time.

Only gradually and reluctantly did we begin to get the hang of this educative process and toe the line – a sort of semi-delinquent dressage. Jennie's approach was a far cry from our flattened hierarchy, consensus decision-making and general 'blurring' psychotherapeutic philosophies and we did not yield them without a struggle. Only slowly therefore did we start to see the sense of Jennie's firm educational approach. It then did become fun, as well as being occasionally frustrating. We felt 'jolly', pausing to indoctrinate a neophyte HDT member to the equestrian's wiles and ways and smiling sadistically at their confusion about 'whats' and 'hows'! Examples might help to illustrate the process and emergent product.

Knowledge and skills

We needed to create a relevant Henderson TC knowledge base. This would have application to all staff in the new services, though would vary, depending on the individual's precise professional role. There would be differing needs for the level of knowledge required according to the particular role within the staff team. For some there was a need to understand the basic TC principles but no need to work the clinical system. (This would apply to some administrative and managerial staff.) Others would need to be able to operate within the therapeutic programme, but not manage it. The most senior clinical staff would not only need to operate the system but also manage it and teach it! The challenge was to try to meet all of the educational needs of the various staff. So we needed to be clear not only about the knowledge base but, as importantly, what were the skills related to operating the model, including its management.

Defining the knowledge base turned out to be easier said than done, as did most tasks associated with this replication project. We had access to the Rapoport study findings and much rhetoric from the early Maxwell Jones writings and had the invigorating literature about TCs in action as well as some in terminal decline (Baron 1987). However, what we could not identify from all of this was the particular knowledge, as opposed to the generic knowledge, that could adequately inform the running of Henderson's democratic TC model in the late 1990s. Generic knowledge relating to the notional or ideal TC would not suffice. Information relating to the setting up of different models of TC might be relevant but we could not use any such, straightforwardly, as precise blueprints or recipes to follow. Both of our new services would require their own unique recipes, though sufficiently similar, which would take account of the actual prevailing conditions within the hosting NHS Trusts and wider community environments where the services were to be located.

Knowledge objectives

The four ideological themes of Rapoport (Rapoport 1960) related to structural elements, such as the democratic voting system and the programme's task-orientated work groups, but also to aspects of 'culture'. These formed the raw material that we needed to blend to construct rateable items linked to knowledge, attitudes and skills. But we also needed to judge what we could reasonably expect staff (we had no new staff at this point) to acquire in the time available, although we did not know what their educational needs were nor how long we actually had to meet these. The amount of time available would be decided by the length of time taken to obtain suitable premises in which to house the new services, as well as the success of our recruitment strategy (see Chapter 5).

With the skilled educational support of Brian Jolly and (especially) the horse-woman Jennie, and after much labour, we generated the following overall training objectives, which were to enable staff to re-negotiate their practitioner roles and specifically to facilitate them to:

- understand the philosophy, culture and structure of the democratic TC
- operate effectively within a flattened staff hierarchy, while maintaining professional boundaries and working with role responsibility
- enable residents' active involvement within the TC
- understand the interplay between socio-therapy and psychotherapy and their importance in the overall treatment model
- be able to impart TC principles and practices to other staff and residents by example and via teaching.

By the end of the training period, therefore, new staff would be expected to have knowledge of:

- history, philosophy and types of TCs
- aetiology of PD, its sub-categorisations and interpersonal effects
- criteria for selection and composition of the resident group
- an authentic treatment alliance as opposed to an illusory alliance
- formal/informal and core/peripheral aspects of the structure
- boundary-setting

- identification of group processes in the informal time
- the interface of the TC with other relevant services and agencies
- the impact of cultural and racial factors on diagnosis, selection and treatment.

These knowledge objectives needed to be translated into relevant skills, including 'masterly inactivity', so that they could be identified within the work situation, by the HDT, when it visited the service once they had been set up.

Turning themes into rateable items

The first step in establishing rateable behaviour items was to identify generic headings capturing the essence of Rapoport's famous four themes. We carried out the task as a group exercise, under strict direction or rather facilitation – the expertise after all was our own, even if we lacked basic discipline in converting our knowledge into identifiable skills. 'Democratisation' seemed the most pertinent place to start for a democratic TC treatment model! This we translated into 'Empowering the Community' and we developed it as follows, into behaviours that we believed could be rated as present or absent:

- deferring to residents in areas where there is a reasonable expectation that they have the requisite knowledge and skills
- allowing time for residents to solve problems or offer suggestions
- facilitating residents in the evaluating and processing of emotional material prior to important decision-making (for example, selection or discharge of residents)
- helping residents to prioritise (for example, distinguishing between urgent and non-urgent business)
- avoiding patronising attitudes and overactive participation, whether in the formal programme or unstructured time
- utilising the 'structure'.

Note that the last of these skills (including skill in using the 'voting' apparatus) was cross-referenced to another skill set – 'Supporting the Therapeutic Structure'. This reflects the fact that some skills are integral to more than one of the ideological themes, hence may belong to more than one set of skills. 'Supporting the Therapeutic Structure', which derived from both the themes of democratisation and reality confrontation, was further unpacked into its associated behaviours, namely:

- maintaining a thoughtful approach to structure
- liaising appropriately with the community's elected senior residents with respect to 'referred meetings'
- maintaining punctual attendance and understanding the importance of time boundaries
- using the opportunities for peer and other supervision, including the 'team awareness' (at the time known as 'sensitivity') meeting
- being aware of the limits of the TC to contain destructively-aroused individuals
- liaising with outside agencies, as appropriate, and especially in regard to discharge.

The process of unpacking the ideological themes and re-configuring them as skills to be acquired, from which there might be observable and rateable behaviours, was not at all straightforward. The process provoked much debate and consternation among us in the HDT, not only because the intellectual activity was unfamiliar but also, importantly, because the nature of the task was complex. Not all the themes lent themselves to the unpacking treatment. 'Permissiveness', for example, proved particularly problematic. In the end, however, it was translated into 'Reflection on and Analysis of the Group' and 'Self-reflection within the Group'. These two skill sets provided the following behaviours that would be looked for during the HDT's visits to the new services. 'Reflection on and Analysis of the Group' gave us:

- responding appropriately within the formal groups and after-groups
- disclosing appropriately a subjective experience of group processes
- suggesting themes arising out of the group experience
- linking issues and themes in the smaller groups to those in the wider community
- making use of formal learning opportunities and supervision
- identifying and resolving inter-staff issues.

'Self-reflection within the Group', very much overlapping and only arbitrarily separate, was translated into:

- recognising destructive group processes which inhibit reflective practice
- identifying learning opportunities through self-reflection
- allowing own emotions to be identified, examined and challenged
- developing reflective practice in relation to learning needs of others.

Agreeing the precise wording for each of these behaviours was also not without its difficulties, and much debate and disagreement was encountered. Frequently the matter would be resolved by subgroups of HDT going off after the expert-led weekly meeting with 'homework', in order to wrestle more privately with the minutiae. Pedantic tendencies, not normally visible to one another in the usual workplace setting, were revealed in those characters least expected to harbour them.

'Communalism' was not easy to translate, perhaps unexpectedly so. At first sight it seemed to represent self-evident behaviour. But our subsequent discussions suggested otherwise. This ideological theme stood for more than simply collaborating to pursue concrete tasks. Eventually, after much labouring, we re-fashioned this into 'Working Constructively with Group Processes'. The skill set had to incorporate a response to perceived defensive acting out or other unhelpful collusion with the more anti-social tendencies of residents (or staff). These skills also related to those of 'Empowering the Community' and hence to the ideological theme of democratisation. Its behaviours are:

- displaying a democratic tendency
- effectively intervening in the face of destructive group processes
- avoiding an overly personalised focus on individuals
- relying on consensus decision-making
- having in mind the context of the group within its wider system(s)
- awareness of impact of culture and race.

This last behaviour clearly relates to the generic skill, rather than solely TC skill, associated with 'Respecting and Supporting Cultural and Racial Difference'. Its component behaviours were identified as:

- awareness of the possible impact of your own culture on those from another culture
- willingness to examine own cultural assumptions, prejudices, preconceived ideas and belief systems
- willingness to explore racial/cultural issues in the resident and staff group
- awareness of the impact of culture and race on assessment, diagnosis and treatment of individuals with mental health problems
- awareness of the need to liaise with outside agencies in order to remove obstacles which may prevent or discourage people from ethnic minorities from joining the community

- respecting the range of backgrounds of all individuals within the therapeutic setting

- demonstrating an understanding of policy and procedures.

Although at times we found the process tedious in the extreme, we also attempted to distil this last 'behaviour' even further, perhaps as a test of the concept of 'reality confrontation'. It is of course important to recognise and value NHS and Trust contexts that necessarily influence the establishment and the maintaining of a culture of enquiry within the clinical arena. Thus 'Understanding Policy and Procedures and Using Them Effectively', as a skill, was distilled as follows:

- being aware of local Trust policy and procedures and ensuring they are taken into account as part of the democratic therapeutic community (DTC) practice

- creating, maintaining and managing appropriate links with relevant external clinical support services

- being aware of mental health legislation and how it impinges on the DTC

- making an appropriate input to the processing of referrals

- taking part in the development of a local marketing strategy

- ensuring that good equal opportunities policy and practice are integrated within the DTC

- ensuring health and safety legislation is operated in line with DTC philosophy

- enabling a good relationship with the local community.

Also on the theme of 'reality confrontation', but closer to its original intended meaning, were the final two sets of skills – 'Managing Professional Boundaries' and 'Integrating Unstructured Time'. Again these skills and the behaviours that would provide evidence that the skill had been acquired were not purely related to the ideological theme that Rapoport and his colleagues had described. But this was not a simple exercise nor one undertaken out of a purely academic interest in how such ideas might be utilised in the service of forming a training agenda or curriculum. We needed to convince ourselves, let alone anyone else, that we had thought and planned enough about both the content and mode of delivery of the training so that we could launch ourselves confidently on the new services with their fledgling TCs. At all costs we wished to avoid coming down too critically on the 'trainees'. We also wanted to provide something of a safety net if they looked like coming a cropper. It would be a tricky business. Formulating and re-formulating these basic ideas, so we believed, would help us in our task and, incidentally, aid HDT to cohere as a group in its unaccustomed educative activity.

'Managing Professional Boundaries' unpacked behaviourally as:

- understanding the therapeutic significance of keeping professional boundaries

- being able to discuss 'boundary' issues and phenomena (e.g. roles in the group, both staff and residents)

- recognising the effect of inappropriate boundary relationships in the development of the personality disordered client group and the impact on professional clinical practice

- modelling appropriate therapeutic boundary behaviour, both in the structured and unstructured time, i.e. respecting others' privacy and rights to confidentiality

- working constructively within professional boundaries in unstructured time and sharing a willingness to examine the impact of these issues on the client group

- reflecting on own boundaries and the effect they have on the interplay in the therapeutic relationship.

'Integrating Unstructured Time' became:

- communicating information from social time to other team members

- willingness to analyse information with the rest of the staff team

- finding a therapeutic way to feed back to residents relevant material from unstructured time

- facilitating residents to feed back to each other material from the unstructured time

- examining one's own behaviour and feelings held during the unstructured time in an attempt to try to understand transference and counter-transference.

The above set of skills, although we had not anticipated it, would turn out to be the most difficult to acquire.

The list of '54' behaviours which we, as HDT, had identified (during the better part of a year's worth of at least weekly meetings) were to have been shared with the trainees. In the event this did not occur since, later on, we concluded that the list might be too daunting or intimidating. Therefore it was re-configured as a checklist for HDT, linked in a grid format with structural elements in the programme (see Table 2.1). Interestingly, although these skill sets did inform the training courses, they never really imparted a strong flavouring to the HDT visits to the new sites. It seemed that the usefulness of the exercise in deriving these 54 behaviours had lain in engendering a strong sense of teamwork in the HDT staff that would stand us in good stead during the long delays we were to encounter! The exercise also served to lessen our dependence on the 'famous four' ideological themes. In the process we all developed a much more complex view of our work that we had hitherto undertaken often intuitively.

Table 2.1 Skills assessment form

	Daily community meetings (with Top 3 chairing)	Referred meetings	Handover (including involvement of residents)	After-groups	Support for staff	Residents actively Involved in the running of the community (including selection and discharge)	Small group therapy	Multi-disciplinary handover	Work groups	Integrated staff group working the rota
Empowering the community										
Reflection on and analysis of the group										
Working constructively with group processes										
Self-reflection within the group										
Integrating unstructured time										
Managing professional boundaries										
Supporting the therapeutic structure										
Understanding policy and procedures and using them effectively										
Respecting and supporting cultural and racial difference										

In a real sense, those of us in HDT had ourselves to become students. We had to confront our own fear about our deficiencies, as well as recognising that we often, with help, had the ability to achieve what at first sight we had not thought possible, namely, to create a relevant syllabus and a feasible teaching method that might work. This sharing of an experience of feeling ignorant but surviving it, we hoped, would help us relate more empathetically to the new staff than we might otherwise have been able to do. In our own experience of supervision, via the expert educationalists, sometimes we had felt supported and enriched by the exercise and sometimes chastised and misunderstood. These and more were to be the responses we evoked from the new staff as we embarked on the training trails to Birmingham and Crewe.

New staff training programme

It was likely, because of the scarcity of democratic TCs in the UK, that few staff recruited would have the requisite skills and experience. Therefore we designed a training strategy whose delivery we hoped would provide what was necessary. It would be delivered via the following processes:

- experiencing the model
- learning about the model
- working the model
- teaching the model.

Experiencing the TC model would be via placements at Henderson. These were envisaged for all the senior staff, but also for some of the more junior posts so that every discipline had at least some members who had experienced the model first hand. This, it was agreed between HDT and our educationalists, would help with flattening the staff hierarchy, since it would not simply be the seniors who were 'in the (TC) know'.

The experience of the placements was to be digested and assimilated during the ensuing day-release training courses. These, it was envisaged, would run in parallel with the carrying out of other tasks and networking/marketing with local professionals and other relevant agencies and resident recruitment. As far as possible this training would mimic the apprenticeship model of incorporating new staff into the Henderson team, although would fall short of this. HDT would visit the new residential TC services during their first 18 months of operation, on a reducing schedule – weekly, fortnightly and monthly – to facilitate learning while actually working in the TC model. The most senior staff would be engaged also in teaching the model, both within the TC and to wider psychiatric and other relevant audiences – also part of 'marketing' the services.

To accelerate the learning process for new staff and to aid them in recruiting potential new residents, current and ex-residents of Henderson were to be prominent in the training role, as members of HDT. Their input would, ideally, complement that of HDT staff members or, if in conflict, could provide opportunities to discuss the meaning and significance of such differences of opinion. Potentially, these discussions would model to the new staff ways of doing business across the usual 'staff–residents' divide, albeit that some members of HDT were ex-residents. Elaborate methods were developed, independently in Birmingham and Crewe, involving HDT – staff and ex-residents – in relation to the task of recruiting residents. At Henderson, residents play a key role in the admission process, through selecting new residents and chairing many of the important meetings, including the daily (Monday to Saturday) meeting of the whole community (see Table 1.1). Ex-residents, having experienced a year in the TC, are well versed in group work and to an extent have some experience of training through welcoming professionals at a weekly visitors' day (part of the established programme) and explaining the workings of the community to them. It was therefore envisaged that they could become involved in the selection of the first cohort of residents in the new services and in some training of the new staff. The aim was to involve, but not overburden, ex-residents. They were to occupy an important but rather limited role.

However, it was soon realised that the ex-residents had much more to contribute than we had given them credit for. In so many ways their knowledge of the TC was superior to ours. They had really lived the experience – 'twenty four/seven' – and as non-resident staff we were mere part-timers by comparison. Therefore a third area was added to the list of roles for ex-resident input, that of 'replication support', i.e. visiting the new units once in operation to see if they were 'getting it right' – to support the trainees' learning from working the model. In the process HDT realised that we needed to be in regular communication with the ex-residents and to recognise their contribution by making them full members of the team. This meant therefore their having a say in the planning, as well as the execution, of the training programme. Ex-residents would therefore be involved in each phase of the training and the HDT would comprise both staff and ex-residents (the latter to become known as 'Volunteers').

Placements

Placements were organised in advance, depending on the educational needs of those visiting, but with certain elements always in common. Thus, all had the same pack of academic papers mailed out in advance. This included, as part of a 'basic papers' pack, seminal papers relating to TCs in general and to Henderson Hospital in particular. The plan was that the visiting professional would read these before arrival so as to avoid being overwhelmed by an experience of novelty that might detract from a useful learning experience. Once on placement there would be opportunities to discuss the content of such papers with other visiting colleagues and with HDT and other Henderson staff.

The essentials of the weekly programme of each placement were similar though tailored according to the nature of the appointment, especially whether it was a 'rota' as opposed to a '9 to 5' staff member. In the case of the latter every effort was made to accommodate the staff members to experience at least one evening of informal time (5 p.m. to 10 p.m.), in addition to the formal parts of the therapeutic programme (8.45 a.m. to 4.45 p.m.), so as to appreciate what their rota staff colleagues might be expected to encounter. Also there was the need to include an important 'shadowing' of duty staff – those who meet with the 'Top Three' residents to establish whether to call an emergency ('referred') meeting – in the case of both nursing staff and social therapists (i.e. rota staff) and of 'surgery' in relation to nursing and medical only.

In practice this meant a lot of programmed activity to include, given that attendance at emergency meetings was also a necessary part of the training programme. Indeed, the placement was meant to be intensive, with as full as possible an immersion in the treatment programme and both formal and informal teaching, from Henderson staff. This was to deepen the trainees' understanding of the 'why' of the TC treatment model. Optimally, new staff would visit with a colleague or two from the same service, partly for social reasons – to make it less burdensome and lonely – but also to promote discussion and greater learning thereby. For reasons beyond HDT's control, this state of affairs was not always realised.

Neither was it possible to arrange for visiting staff placements to be timed at the convenience of the Henderson. It had been envisaged that there would be a system of 'two weeks on and two weeks off', so that Henderson could recover regularly from having visitors on such an intensive basis and over a prolonged period. Delays to recruitment in the new services, however, would mean that the planned spread of visits could not occur. The resultant cramming would mean that there was increasingly a feeling of Henderson being invaded – increasingly resented by both residents and staff. This resulted in a loss of goodwill and a lessening of the informal time spent with staff, hence a relative loss of one key ingredient of the programme – informal inter-staff contact and learning.

It was also the case that some staff were given concrete tasks to achieve by their managers, over and above that of simply imbibing the democratic TC model, for example, obtaining details of Henderson's food preparation and kitchen hygiene policies – we did not have either one! What were these? In the view of HDT, this multi-tasking obscured the main task and as a consequence diminished the value of the placement. In spite of this, the feedback from these 'visitors' tended to be positive. To an extent, however, this depended on aspects peripheral to the placement, such as the degree to which colleagues bonded with one another out of hours! The quality of accommodation seemed also to play a part, and an attempt to cut costs by using lower-quality accommodation backfired. We concluded that damp and mouldy accommodation neither encour-

Table 2.2 Weekly programme for core staff

WEEK 1 – CORE STAFF (9–5)

		MONDAY	TUESDAY	WEDNESDAY	THURSDAY	FRIDAY
8.50–9.10 a.m.	Handover	✓	✓	✓		✓
9.15–10.30	Community meeting	✓	✓	✓		✓
10.35–10.50	Review	✓	✓	✓		✓
11.00–12.15	AM groups	Introduction to placement	Teaching	Teaching		New residents
12.15–1.00 p.m.				LUNCH		
1.00–2.00	Staff meeting	✓	✓	✓	✓	✓
2.15–4.30	PM group	Teaching	Selection/ Unit reception	Teaching	Work group 1	Work group 1
4.30–10.00	Social time				✓	
	Supper				✓	
	Summit meeting				✓	

WEEK 2 – CORE STAFF (9–5)

		MONDAY	TUESDAY	WEDNESDAY	THURSDAY	FRIDAY
8.50–9.10 a.m.	Handover	✓	✓	✓	✓	✓
9.15–10.30	Community meeting	✓	✓	✓	✓	✓
10.35–10.50	Review	✓	✓	✓	✓	✓
11.00–12.15	AM groups	New residents	Teaching	New residents	Teaching	New residents
12.15–1.00 p.m.		LUNCH				
1.00–2.00	Staff meeting	✓	✓	✓	✓	✓
2.15–4.30	PM group	Teaching	Selection/Unit reception	Teaching	Work group 2	Work group 2
4.30–10.00 p.m.	Social time				✓	
	Supper				✓	
	Summit meeting				✓	

aged learning nor the enjoyment of training and we did not repeat that experiment – sorry, Michael.

Eventually, in July 2000, as the week-on-week placements had taken their toll, notice was given that they could no longer be sustained. We stopped them. This was experienced as an abrupt cessation, in spite of a month's notice having been given and it gave rise to resentment from the two new services' staff teams and Directors. HDT felt the new services' staff failed to appreciate how draining these placements had been on the 'parent' Henderson. Maybe the weaning period was too short, although no individual staff member was in fact prematurely detached from the Henderson breast! Rather, those last in post were deprived of the placements they might have been expecting. This represented one of a number of low points in the replication project.

The day release course

Unexpected obstacles, mainly arising from the difficulty in recruiting to order in the two new services, meant that the originally planned day release courses in fact ran only once and had to metamorphose (at very short notice) into residential courses. The latter were held on two occasions, and, on account of time constraints, both close together and also close to the actual opening times of the new services (September 2000). This was counter to the original idea of having time in between the training events, i.e. a day release model of delivery that would support the gradual, hence more thoughtful, assimilation of the learning, so that it could be more informative of the clinical work. This would be effected via the setting of 'homework' – tasks to be undertaken between the weekly sessions. Indeed, this was the format of the first course and the feedback from it for new staff was good. However, even then, the composition of the membership was not ideal, being an unequal distribution between the two services' staff. The main aims had been to maximise learning, not to build teams, and to build some sense of unity among the three staff teams that would comprise this single national severe PD service.

The day release course, through highlighting important aspects of the therapy programme, would reinforce the observational learning that had been derived from the placements. This would be achieved through discussion (disagreement, if necessary) and via a thorough exploration of issues in a forum that included 'experts by experience' – some of Henderson's ex-service users. The topics for the training days related to the skill sets described earlier:

- personality disorder/therapeutic community
- authentic and illusory alliances
- integrating unstructured time
- managing professional boundaries

- respecting and supporting cultural differences
- formal and informal structure and culture
- supporting therapeutic structure and culture
- leadership and role definition within a flattened hierarchy.

Placements were only ever envisaged as one part of the learning process, since it was acknowledged that there would be a steep learning curve for many new staff. Henderson was a tertiary service – most referrals hailing from psychiatrists – and only a few of those recruited to each new service had worked in such specialised settings before. Also, no matter how skilled they might be individually, all would need to learn how to work alongside one another, as part of a new team, in a wide range of group settings. They would need to understand how their own role related to those of a range of colleagues, some from similar and some from different professional backgrounds. The purpose of the training courses was thus also to help embed the model into the 'teams'. (It was recognised that actual team-building would be primarily the remit of the Local Implementation Teams – the local counterpart to the HDT – and the relevant senior staff (trainers) from the new services.) Role-play was to figure prominently to complement learning via traditional academic seminars. Additional ex-service users would join the HDT to deliver the training on these courses. Their involvement was not merely tokenistic (see above and Ormrod and Norton 2003).

Table 2.3 gives an indication of the evaluation and feedback of the '5 weeks of 2 days each' post-placement day release courses (it derives from the first day of the first course – on personality disorder and therapeutic community). The numbers attending the course fluctuated, from 10 to 15 out of a possible total of 15 staff, and with an average of 12. The tenth day was set up as a day whose programme was to be organised by the delegates/trainees themselves. It was not rated by them. Feedback was collected anonymously, and space was provided for

Table 2.3 Evaluation of relevance – Course 1, Day 1 (2 May 2000)

	Highly relevant	Mostly relevant	Of little relevance	Not at all relvant
Pre-info	7	5		
10.00 a.m.–11.00 a.m.	5	9		
11.30 a.m.–12.45 p.m.	6	6		
1.30 p.m.–2.45 p.m.	5	6	2	
3.00 p.m.–3.45 p.m.	4	9		
Overall	4	7		
Total	**31**	**42**	**2**	**0**

trainees to comment in writing, in addition to ticking the relevant boxes, regarding how relevant they had found the training. There was also an opportunity to share verbal comments at the end of each training day with the whole group in the 3–3.45 p.m. session. Using this range of methods we attempted to obtain as much feedback as possible, which we would use to refine subsequent courses. The length of the study day was relatively short for two reasons, one theoretical, the other practical. The idea was that the course should be enjoyable as well as relevant. Some of the delegates and all of HDT had to travel to Birmingham on the morning of Day 1 and from Birmingham to Euston, London on the second day.

HDT kept a record of how the course was delivered and we recorded our views in a 'collective diary'. Our comments on the first day of the first course, framed more as questions, were as follows:

?   *tolerating 'not knowing' a problem – evidenced by overtly reasonable request for more information, especially with respect to PD theory*

?   *ambivalence about Henderson Hospital personnel (as 'staff' – versus residents)*

?   *sufficient knowledge base provided*

?   *author (of one of the papers) present*

?   *new/junior, old/senior 'split'*

?   *more process than content*

It had been the suggestion of our educationalist consultants that the trainees and the trainers should mix socially, staying overnight in a local hotel, following a communal meal after the first day of the course. This we did, although not all the trainees availed themselves of this or were able to attend due to personal or family reasons. (This should be borne in mind given our record of the next day of the course.) The idea was to facilitate learning through speeding up the processes of cohesion within this group of adult learners, most of whom already worked together (though there was little or no 'clinical' work at this early stage). It should also be noted that in mingling socially, trainees and trainers would be eroding the conventional hierarchical relationship that exists between them – an aspect in harmony with the democratic TC ideology.

HDT's comments in respect of Day 2 of the course – 'Authentic and illusory treatment alliances' – recognised that some trainees seemed to be occupying marginal positions within the group for reasons that were not clear. We had concerns about the social event of the previous evening – that it might not have had the desired effect. Some staff, we noted, were very new to their posts. For one member, this course represented the first and second days of employment! This individual had had no time to be inducted. A difficult (local management) decision had been made to include rather than exclude the person from the course. The latter option would have been particularly problematic since the course was situated in the workplace – for reasons of financial economy – so there would have been nowhere else for this member to go. Delaying taking up the position by the five weeks that the course covered had been an option but the potential for getting to know the team and getting up to speed with the training was, in the end, deemed more of an opportunity to be grasped than a threat. (Interestingly, this staff member was the first to leave the service, though this was some 18 months later.)

It was noted by HDT that the new staff seemed be 'hearing it from ex-residents' (i.e. seemed to understand it better than from them than from HDT staff), including what the staff's duties should and should not be! Compared to that of the first day, the overt academic content appeared to be grappled with more successfully – 'process *and* content' was the note. We wondered whether there should be a greater ex-resident input, given the more positive reception of their ideas – not palpably different in content compared to our own. (N.B. Ex-residents were involved only in the second day of each two-day block.) We wondered whether more time should be allowed in the programme for the discussion of papers circulated beforehand and also whether written prompts should accompany these in order to identify the key learning points.

We felt there was still some reticence among the new staff about demonstrating their knowledge (or ignorance) in front of the group, some of which would be within the realms of what is 'normal'. Feedback from the trainees themselves had indicated that they had appreciated the relative lack of didactic approach. However, some felt that the ex-residents were too active. Some felt perturbed by HDT occupying different roles within the day, at times taking up participative roles, and at other times more observer or reflective roles. We had an elaborate arrangement, whereby there was an HDT Chair for the course, a Large Group Convenor for the last meeting of each day – during which feedback on that day was collected – and also Theme Convenors who each had responsibility for organising the particular day's topic! Why did we do it that way? My recollection is that this was to avoid locating the leadership function within a single individual – hence modelling functional leadership, as an aspect of hierarchy flattening.

Much of this course was fun. The HDT, in travelling together by train from Euston to Birmingham, would use the time to plan/fine tune the course during the journey, based on the previous week's feedback. Much of this was in fact (unusually for this project) going according to plan. We did feel under pressure to get it right, however, since we knew there would be no second chance. We recognised that some of our anxiety about performing well as trainers probably mirrored that of the trainees who did not know if they could deliver a therapeutic community in the near future. We thought it an example of 'parallel processes'. This was May 2000 and the TCs were thought to be opening in July, although later it was decided, by each independently, that opening in the middle of the holiday season would be silly.

HDT found itself worrying about the group process during the training days and also whether the 'right' new staff had been appointed. Thus, at times we would be concerned that a particular member would not be able to stand up to the rigours of TC work based on his or her performance at this course. The situation was even more complicated by the fact that some of those attending were doing so with their line managers! But this, after all, had been our intention – in the interests of 'flattening' hierarchies. If we had worries about a particular individual trainee, how would we deal with these? At what point would we be obliged to make a formal statement to a line manager? These anxieties, although having some basis in fact and being no different from the proper concerns of any who put on training, exercised us prominently. We should probably have anticipated this. We wondered if these were further examples of parallel processing – questions that the new staff were (unconsciously) asking about one another's suitability.

So, this first course was not all plain sailing. At the beginning of the third week, one of the senior staff attending questioned the relevance of the course now that it was known that, because of a delay in recruitment, the opening of the services would be delayed. The introduction of this note of doubt over the course's value may have been responsible for the moans that there was too much for trainees to do, in addition to attending the course, given the imminence of the opening. They also felt that some of us spoke too much and in 'paragraphs rather than sound bites'! Who were they talking about? We think we knew.

'Respecting and supporting difference', Day 6, was felt by some to be a difficult experience. We caused possible confusion by inviting local new staff to lead on this as Theme Convenors – since we did not consider this to be HDT's strong suit. Maybe this was an error, since it demanded much of the rest of the trainees to re-orientate both to their colleagues' sudden change of status and role (as trainers) and to that of the HDT membership – we joined in with them as if trainees too. We were in fact embodying a core principle of TCs which dictates that expertise should be recognised wherever it resides. Overall we felt it to have been a successful and participative day. One positive comment received was that the ex-residents also seemed to be 'on a level playing field'.

Day 7 saw the complex relationship between the TC's 'structure and culture' addressed and unpacked. Role-play was a very prominent aspect of this day's training. It was felt that the scenarios chosen had been relevant but that the time allowed for their unpacking was too short. Some of the day had been, possibly, 'too cerebral'. There was little feedback on what had transpired with more (avoidant) focus on what was to happen the following day. It was clear from feedback on the next day of the course that we had indeed assumed far too much knowledge about Henderson's structures, in spite of the fact that many trainees had experienced week-long (or longer) placements. This realisation was too late to benefit those attending but would be borne in mind by HDT for the two future courses. It was also felt that to reverse the order of Days 7 and 8 would have brought more coherence. There seemed to be a difference in level of activity, perhaps related to confidence/knowledge of the DTC, between those who had already visited and those who had not – a relief that there was evidence of benefit from the placements!

Day 9 explored 'Leadership and role definition', though it was interesting that at short notice two of the most senior staff attending were unavoidably absent. It was not clear in what ways this might have affected what took place. Some difficult issues emerged, regarding gender, sexism and 'sexual tensions'. In a role-play there had been mention of 'an affair with the leader' – possibly from the depths of the delegates' unconscious, perhaps out of mischief! Our notes state that there was not much disagreement among the trainees but that there were 'undercurrents'!

The final day had been promising to be a disaster given the prior reluctance of most to entertain what was planned. This was for the members to organise their own programme. This had been a tried and tested ingredient of the Henderson's Groupwork Course, very successfully run over many years to multi-disciplinary and multi-agency audiences from within the NHS and outside. They had tended to be highly creative during this day of the course. Perhaps this was by virtue of being strangers to one another at least at the start and having little likelihood of meeting one another again in the future. The situation in Birmingham was clearly different. Although we had some relative strangers, most had been working and would continue to work closely with each other. There might also have been rivalry between the two new staff teams themselves and/or with ourselves, as future colleagues. So, how did the day go?

A budget, not generous but a budget nevertheless had been provided (£50). With this had been purchased a range of art materials. The event surprised all in the extent to which it was actually collaborative. The idea had been to form three subgroups and for each (graphically) to depict a TC. The results were not artistic, nor obviously informative, but it was the process more than the product which was important. To me the ex-residents had seemed marginal to the process, but nonetheless they reported feeling positively affected and involved (as they revealed to HDT staff in our joint after-group with them). In the final afternoon feedback session, suggestions for improving the course and other ideas for subsequent courses emerged. HDT were congratulated on our commitment to the course. Concern was expressed that most of the social therapists were being recruited late and that this could have (or was already having) a marginalising effect within the new staff teams. Disturbingly, themes of 'decapitation' and the 'origin of oxygen' arose in the final large group feedback session. (We wondered to ourselves what effect the organisational researcher's presence might have contributed but did not feel this was likely to have been sufficient to generate the fantasy of decapitation!).

Table 2.4 gives the total feedback for this first course in terms of daily totals.

Table 2.4 Evaluation of relevance – Course 1 daily totals

Day	Highly relevant	Mostly relevant	Of little relevance	Not at all relevant
1	31	42	2	
2	32	25	1	
3	57	13		
4	26	45	1	
5	37	23		
6	33	14	1	
7	33	30		
8	34	17	2	
9	17	29	2	

TC vignettes

To give a further flavour of the course, it might be informative to describe the vignettes or scenarios that we enacted during the training. These role-play exercises were directed by Henderson staff trained in psychodrama or drama-therapy who had experience of undertaking this work with Henderson clients. Therefore they had relevant credentials for this aspect of the training, which tended to go down very well with the trainees, perhaps being more palatable than the lectures and seminars. Maybe this was a medium that was less revealing, or at least revealing of a different aspect of the trainees' professional or personal selves. Maybe it lessened the divide between the more senior/managerial and those who had to deal with the actual nitty-gritty of the front-line work. Maybe it appealed simply to the more extroverted.

THE PATIO DOORS

At night the security of Henderson Hospital is maintained, in part, through a tour of the building by one duty staff member and one resident. On the night in question, two residents asked to remain outside on the patio, saying they would lock the doors after they came inside. The 'night round' staff member said this was not acceptable since she had responsibility, along with the senior resident, for securing all outside doors. Both 'patio' residents were verbally abusive to the staff member. The resident member kept silent.

When next in a community meeting the issue was revisited by the verbally abused staff member and a similar argument ensued. Later, in staff supervision, a heated argument broke out concerning what was the right course of action to take in this circumstance. Whose responsibility was it to lock the doors at night – staff or residents? Could authority be delegated to residents?

The enactment of this vignette soon generated a head of steam, as the soon-to-be TC staff found themselves in hot debate. The issue of delegation of staff power and authority strikes at the heart of the matter of empowering the resident subgroup. Delegates could imagine how in practice it might not be clear just where to draw the line, even when it concerned an aspect as important as the security of the building. This vignette also revealed something of the tensions that exist between the different ideological themes. In this instance it was the issue of 'communalism' (i.e. shared and collaborative working together to make the place safe at night) and 'permissiveness'. The tension between these two themes needed to be managed, since the two potentially collaborating parties – staff and residents – did not agree on a concerted way forward.

The vignette also served to highlight how similar arguments and issues become echoed around different forums, sometimes appearing within the wider community and at times within a particular subgroup of it – here the staff team subgroup. Issues are seldom 'black and white' in nature, so it is less whether authority can be delegated and more how much of it can, under what circumstances, and to whom. Importantly it is the thinking, verbalising and the fact of the discussions about the issue – the process – that is required of the democratic TC model rather than the actual outcome. This represents the enactment of a 'culture of enquiry' (see Norton 1992).

THE VOTE

Henderson's community was tired. Senior staff were frequently absent for a variety of reasons – new services development, maternity leave, sickness. Some staff felt the existing management structures had been outgrown and suggested the need for external management restructuring advice. Part of the latter entailed finding more time for staff to meet. This situation was shared with the residents at the time.

Later, the plans for change were announced following consultation with the residents. The proposed change to the Wednesday programme proved unpopular, even though the prior discussion with residents had been productive. At the implementation of this change, the main senior staff negotiator was off sick. The change went ahead but the residents were not happy. They felt disempowered and 'conned'.

Outreach staff (involved in the change to the Wednesday programme) became the target of scapegoating. They were challenged to name all the residents in the community, which they agreed they could not do! The resident chair of the meeting proposed they should therefore forfeit their vote. After some discussion this motion was carried with some (residential) staff support. Outreach staff felt betrayed, especially by their residential colleagues. Who could let this happen?

Again, as with the earlier vignette, the issue of power was to the fore. Who should have it, and under what circumstances, according to the democratic TC model, can it be delegated? There was clearly a difference of opinion between the staff and residents as to who could remove the voting rights – a distempering of staff dynamic. But the situation was more complicated, since some staff also agreed with the resident chair's proposal to disenfranchise their colleagues in 'Outreach'. At this point in time, i.e. at the time of the actual events that took place, there was a feeling of 'us' and 'them' among the staff team. The Outreach members were relatively new and strangers and, as such, not fully trusted. Part-timers to the model had always tended to be treated with suspicion – like newcomers to a far-flung village, 'foreigners' until they have lived there 30 years! Secretly, or not so secretly, staff were relieved to see their newer colleagues given short shrift. The implication of the removal of the voting right meant that the staff division was revealed for all to see, and this brought with it an imperative to work on healing this potentially dangerous rift. This vignette exposed the new staff to something of the power of such 'splitting' processes and to its inevitability.

The next course – the first residential course

The plan had been to re-run the '5 x 2-days' training for the rest of the staff as they were recruited. On this basis, refinements (or more major changes) could be made to the courses that followed, leading to improvements and a closer fit between what was needed and provided. Sadly, this was not to be. Delays in re-cruitment, mostly brought about by the delay in finding and refurbishing the new services' premises, meant that if all staff were to receive at least some training this would have to be done within a much shorter time frame. The result was that a hastily revised and reconstructed residential course was designed to achieve two main aims (not one, as previously). The new aim was to provide some 'team-building' in addition to familiarising staff with the most pertinent issues that they might encounter early on in the TC work. Unfortunately, this format could not permit a gradual and gentle reflection on what was taught with homework tasks to support this. Rather, it was a cramming-course – a basic TC survival kit. To achieve this end we launched bigger guns (other senior staff, used to training though not previously engaged with HDT), realising that for some this cramming and pressurised course could prove intimidating and thus backfire. Again, we decided to feature role-play and involve ex-residents extensively in the delivery. Once more we were entering uncharted territory, since little seemed to be going exactly to plan. But by now we had more confidence in our own educational abilities and the value of ex-residents, who had decided by this time that they would prefer to be known as 'Volunteers'. They were now our not-so-secret weapons. And they did not let us down.

Other things did. Some of them were of our own making or at least potentially under our own control. But as recorded in the 'collective diary' on the evening of the first crash course, it was one 'catalogue of blunders', though not all ours. Sadly, one member scheduled to attend was absent due to having to attend a funeral. We had no reason to doubt the authenticity of this reason for absence but we were considerably paranoid by this stage. Rooms in the medium-priced, slightly down-market Surrey hotel were not available for occupation until 4.15 p.m. This heralded a later than advertised start – not a good one.

Then we discovered that too few bedrooms had been reserved. Some were therefore to be 'doubled up' (and not from laughter), for the following night. Also, so we discovered, there had been problems with the mailing out of papers that needed to be read prior to the start of the course – 'pre-information'. This meant that the first session planned had to be substantially reconfigured, in the absence of the paper having been read. So, instead of presenting and discussing a paper on therapeutic community and personality disorders (and in addition to the domestic notices – delivered more slowly and distinctly than was usual, in order to fill the time) we outlined the model of learning that had been chosen. This was in the belief that this might aid digestion of the material to be absorbed and, not least, fill what was felt to be an uncomfortable gap on a Sunday evening away from families and loved ones.

We introduced a 'case vignette', which was to be the meat in the sandwich, but not the whole meal. The new staff were divided into two groups for this exercise. Afterwards they came together to pool thoughts in a large group of all attending. Following this was a 25-minute period of reflection to consider 'Structure and culture', the theme of the next day's study. Feedback from the earlier course had suggested that we had assumed too much of the new staff in terms of familiarity with the way these terms were applied to a therapeutic setting. This was, perhaps, an interesting observation in itself, but we needed to address it pragmatically, given the brief to fast-track. To cap it all the feedback forms that should have been circulated beforehand had not been, so our claim that we took seriously trainees' feedback comments was unconvincing.

Of course, we had an after-group for those of us hapless individuals responsible for the shambles – maybe we should have retired immediately to the bar as we suspected many of the delegates had done. But one of us had a view that the makeshift introduction to the course might have been a more sensible way to start than the way we had planned – to jump in at the deep end with a paper and discussion. Our earlier experience of the 5 x 2 days course had been that some trainees appeared to feel unskilled or under-confident about putting their views to others in a large group setting. Some were complete strangers to one another, many may have resented the loss of a weekend day to attend a 'work' function, and all had made long journeys.

There had been some confusion during the case vignette exercise, due to the fact that the paper (which some had received and read) also included case vignettes, one of which was similar to the one verbally presented to the two groups. Apparently some had brought in details from the written version erroneously. We felt, in our hypersensitive state, that we were picking up some antipathy to the Henderson model. However, we might have misperceive what was (indirect) criticism of our organisational skills. For whatever reason, the notes written in the collective diary for the remainder of the course are sparse. Perhaps HDT were feeling tired and strained. Perhaps we had had enough of things not going according to plan with the project as a whole. Perhaps we had reached the limits of our ingenuity and resourcefulness. At this point we were almost three years into the project proper.

Monday dawned (the first full day of the course) and the ex-residents joined us at the coffee break at 11 a.m. They led an impromptu session on what had been important aspects of the model for them while in treatment. It was chastening for those of us HDT staff who worked '9 to 5' to hear that we were somewhat shadowy and faceless individuals, for the most part only dimly remembered, and that the 'rota staff' tended to be recalled as distinct people in their own right. Well, it was good for flattening the staff hierarchy, as well as that between the course organisation and the delegates! Role-playing figured as the major educational tool for the day. The two Theme Convenors had training in psychodrama and drama-therapy respectively. It is recorded that there was a reflective space from 3 to 3.45 p.m. before a time for private study and reflection – 4 to 5 p.m. No mention of content was made and my memory fails to fill in the gap. Perhaps this is just as well, since the final note in the diary for that Monday was to say that 'admin support was inadequate'.

Tuesday was 'Leadership and role definition' and a paper (Whiteley 1986) by my predecessor, Dr Stuart Whiteley, was to be discussed. It would highlight the cycle of social interaction in the TC, during which inevitable tensions are created and, in dealing with these, emotional and interpersonal difficulties are encountered. All of this is grist to the mill of the small group sessions within the formal programme and also the reason for calling emergency meetings of the whole community. Exploration of antecedents and consequences of such manifest difficulties followed, with new coping strategies identified that can be experimented with during the social time in between formal group meetings, during the evenings and at weekends – at least that is the theory. We then rolled out our two trusty vignettes – 'The patio doors' and 'The vote'. There is no specific diary entry to prompt and I am not sure how these were received on this occasion and from this distance, another three years on.

The 'Pins and straws' exercise was a much more memorable event altogether. We borrowed it from the field of industry, where it had been a tried and tested method with which to explore, in staff teams or among applicants for jobs, attitudes towards leadership and team-playing. At least that was the use to which we put it. The idea is that different leadership styles are assigned to selected individuals (who are designated to take on a leadership role for that project), one per group, without the rest of the group being aware of the style. The three styles were laissez faire, dictatorial and democratic. The teams then, under their leaders, complete the same task building a structure using only 'pins and straws'. At the end of the allotted time, there is discussion of how it felt to be working under the different leadership regimes and also how it felt to be leading.

To our surprise, since some had utilised this device before, it drew some extreme reactions, especially regarding its apparent lack of scientific validity, and hence the justification for its place on the course. The task for each group had been to build the most extravagant but durable structure possible with the time allotted. If the exercise had run true to form, the result should have shown at least marginal advantages to the democratic leadership and, preferably, a decisive superiority. In fact, the nominated leaders' ambivalence in engaging with the task meant that not only was there no clear supremacy of democracy – hence a central plank of our TC model was missing – but also little enjoyment of the task.

We wondered in our after-group whether some staff were feeling marginalised within their new staff groups and whether those who occupied solitary posts within their team might be especially vulnerable. We did not know, nor did we have enough information on which to draw to conclude definitively. Otherwise, we noted that there seemed to be 'life' in the delegates, albeit some of it carrying a distinct negative charge. Part of the teemed day was to spend a limited budget, as a group, on supper, rather than merely descending to the hotel's restaurant. Some were perplexed by the prospect, not thinking this exercise could enrich learning (and perhaps believing it to be further evidence of HDT's nonsensical training strategy). As HDT, we merely indicated that we would 'await feedback'. So we did. And it was surprisingly positive.

The next day's theme was 'Supporting cultural and other differences'. As with the earlier course, the Theme Convenors for this day were to have come from one of the new services, since they seemed better placed than those of us from the HDT, by virtue of being from minority cultures. Maybe this was again a mistake. Perhaps we should have learnt from our experience of the first course. We had believed that we had some grounds for optimism in handing over responsibility for the whole day, not least since the session had been 'rehearsed' in the first course. Non-attendance of the external convenors, however, required last-minute replacements. One of these was the totally reliable Project Manager – Richard Bulmer – who had done much to carry the flag of 'ethnicity' and 'equal ops' throughout the project.

A handout was hastily produced, which outlined the structure for the day with pointed questions being asked, such as 'Who am I?' A pairing exercise appeared to go well, with those attending meeting as couples, for five minutes, for each to tell the other, in most cases a relative stranger, who they were. (This exercise also involved the ex-residents and represented a breaking down of some of the previously well-protected personal–professional boundaries.) The 'couples' then selected issues, such as feeling stigmatised by being from a certain social class or ethnic group to feed back to the rest of the group, from those that had surfaced for them during the brief conversations. Following this, breaking into smaller groups, the course considered other questions in relation to a case vignette, based on a real incident during the unstructured part of the programme when a Henderson resident had made what a staff member considered to be a racist statement. The main question was 'How would the delegates deal with a similar scenario were this to occur in their new TC?'

The day seemed to be going very smoothly, especially considering the shaky start and last minute stand-ins, when the issue of confidentiality in relation to the material aired was raised. This set the scene for a collective paranoid (hysterical?) reaction, as some pondered aloud anxieties about who might get to know what. This anxiety then escalated when a senior member indicated that they held line management responsibility for some of those present and that this responsibility continued during any work-related activity, including this very course! In our HDT after-group it was suggested that some of the anxiety might have been in anticipation of the more senior HDT staff, including myself, being absent for the following day's programme, though this may have been projected anxiety from those who considered themselves junior who had to 'act up'.

The next day was to be 'Being real and therapeutic'. This title derived from a paper written by two of Henderson's social therapists (Juliet Revel and Antonia Reay), one of whom was a member of HDT and due to present it as Theme Covenor. Two other Social Therapists and a Charge Nurse joined her. All were well practised in working during the unstructured times – at weekends and evenings.

As I was not present at this day I can only rely on the written record of those who were to describe what happened. There was said to be a high level of anxiety in the large group that met to discuss the paper, via a traditional seminar approach. The discussion found itself in the territory of 'getting it wrong'. 'People' (meaning the prospective residents in the new services) might kill themselves. It was apparently not at all clear whence this anxiety arose, although the previous day had ended on a similarly anxious note. It was reported that some of the ex-residents teaching on the programme had been concerned lest the new services did not 'get it right' and HDT had a view that they might have sounded overly critical. The role-plays, however, seemed to provide some 'relief and understanding'. Apparently, they helped to allay anxieties through 'putting things into perspective'. It was noted that it was the more junior staff attending the course who seemed to be more willing to admit their anxieties and concerns about therapeutic practice. HDT staff commented in the report (possibly not to the delegates) that the male trainees were appearing 'strong and macho'.

During the after-groups of HDT staff, it was conjectured that the day might have been improved had the ex-residents participated for the whole time. (For a variety of reasons, this had not been the structure set up. Some of these reasons may have been defensive and some paternalistic. The arrangement for their involvement in the entire course was to be present on alternate days and to arrive at the coffee break, after the academic presentation, and also to leave before the reflective larger group at the end of the day.) HDT, on this day, also thought that had the ex-residents been present, the discussion would have been less open among the staff – so maybe the organisation was appropriate after all. There was a lot of performance anxiety around and not just in the delegates! HDT certainly had a lot invested in helping and facilitating the new staff to make our shared enterprise of replication a success. None of us knew if we were up to it. How could we know?

The final reflective space at the end of the day uncovered a number of issues. Living together in close proximity in the hotel resonated with an experience of what it might be like to reside in a TC, where it was not possible to get away – to find the usual amount of privacy and freedom – from colleagues. The influence of my own absence was discussed, apparently, perhaps because I had been so closely identified with the whole replication and training processes for so long. But maybe this was also because the HDT team were without their usual 'leader'. Anyhow, the issue of leaders, and what it felt like when they were not around, was aired, and the session ended with the notion that it was allowable to 'get it wrong' and for that not to be a hanging offence. The course closed the next day at lunchtime and there seemed to be an acknowledgement, at least among us in HDT, that it had been 'good enough'. We would have a break, it being mid-July, before repeating the course in August and just prior to the new services opening in September 2000.

The last course – the second residential course

Not especially refreshed by our respective vacations, HDT were back to work with our final post-placement course – this was only a matter of weeks away from opening. For reasons that escape me and are not elsewhere recorded, I was absent for the first day – Sunday late afternoon – of this last course. Our Project Manager had set out the housekeeping aspects of the course before handing over to the two Theme Convenors for the day, our training lead (Chris Scanlon) and one of the mainstays of the Social Therapists (Kevin Polley) involved with HDT. Following established educational principles the delegates were led through their hopes and fears for the forthcoming course. This enabled discussion of how the course might be modified, even at this late stage, to fulfil hopes and allay fears. It is reported that some attending had appeared not to have read the previously circulated paper – 'TCs and personality disorder'. But the smaller group discussions of the case vignettes drew a more enthusiastic response and positive contribution. In particular, there was debate over how 'safe' the TC model might be compared to more traditional psychiatric models. It is not clear from the notes whether or how this debate was concluded, i.e. whether one or other was considered to be superior or safer. It was noted, as follows: 'how safe is TC to deal with PD and how unsafe traditional models are'. In the HDT after-group there was a questioning of how much (or how little) there was of an understanding of PD but a view that this had been a good first day. Evaluation forms, it is reported, were circulated 'in something of a crush' – no further elaboration!

It was time to be 'real and therapeutic' again. No wonder we were beginning to feel exhausted. We commented on the success of the day only very briefly, via our reflective diary, summarising it as an 'excellent day'. We had, so we congratulated ourselves, discovered the 'final format' for discussing and presenting the role-plays – not before time and arguably a bit late in the day, given this was the last course we would stage. These role-plays had been apt and generated good-quality discussion. Anxieties were raised, however, regarding risk assessment and management that served, in our estimation, to distract from the theme of the day.

We in HDT were at this point concentrating on refining our training technique and prowess and were perhaps insufficiently sensitive to the proximity of the opening and the very real anxieties in the delegates regarding the managing of the situations which were outlined in the vignettes. It was understandable, with hindsight, that anxiety would have been high, and spending more time on going over how the relevant Henderson structures unpacked in terms of assessing and managing risk would have been appropriate. To an extent there could be seen to be a clash of cultures with Henderson's 'historical' culture (rooted in its patient-centred approach and collective methods of dealing with crises) and the new staff's 'modern' culture, perhaps based on risk-aversion and staff-protective policies. Certainly this territory would prove to be one of a number of future battlegrounds to be played out along different frontiers, most notably between the service and its commissioners, but also in the 'replication meetings' (see Chapter 4).

Having been 'real and therapeutic', if also a bit anxious, we were once more into 'Structure and culture', as applied to the TC setting. In our experience of the three courses, this 'day' seemed to generate the greatest difficulty with grasping even the basic concepts – ones we had taken too much for granted and so were inadequately taught. Maybe there were other reasons too, perhaps linked to the other lay meanings attached to the terms or to an unfamiliarity with sociological, as opposed to medical, constructs. We shall never know now, but this was a difficult morning on the course, with one of the Volunteers being also visibly upset, the reasons again were not and are not clear.

For a number of us it was approaching the end of a phase in the project and I guess we had some sense of resignation that it would now be too late to make much of a difference. Perhaps it was related to this that the Volunteer had been upset. Perhaps the Volunteers in their training role appeared more robust than they otherwise were. It was becoming clearer to HDT that there was a difference between running an existing 'elderly' service with experienced staff (i.e. that which HDT knew about) and attempting to set up a new service with staff who hardly knew one another and were mainly novices at the TC method and its application. In the social activities that ensued for course members that evening, there was a minor accident, which had, what was felt at the time to be, a disproportionately large emotional reaction in the remainder of the delegates (and probably on the HDT membership too). It was as if it signified how brittle and fragile were the team relationships in relation to the scale of the replication task! Was this sprain a portent? If so, was the bruising merely superficial or indicative of deeper pathology?

'Respecting and supporting cultural difference' came next. The day included an exercise, borrowed from another course, I believe. This necessitated us all to wear bin-liners (as outer garments) and to have labels, which we ourselves could not read, by virtue of their being on our backs. Others could read them, and the idea of the 'play' was for all to respond to the label rather than to the person. The main aim was to elucidate who it was that the others saw us to be, and via this to feel the tension between being oneself and being responded to as if one were otherwise. This was kind of unfamiliar territory for most of us, kind of uncomfortable and ultimately not necessarily all that edifying once we discussed matters afterwards – also part of the exercise. Some felt it had turned out to be more about boundary-keeping than respecting difference. However, the fact that so many were discomforted and the fact that we could, by virtue of ethnic backgrounds, be naïve to relevant issues, meant that the exercise could have hit the target or at least part of it. Overall, however, our sense was that the issue had generated more heat than light. There was little sharing of issues to do with 'difference' and HDT wondered if the presence of a large number of relatively senior staff among the delegates attending had inhibited openness. Perhaps it was simply the presence of a 'white' majority which exerted this powerful effect.

Conclusions

Not much had gone according to plan from the Henderson's standpoint. The recovery period between visiting staff placements had been obliterated and this strained the TC's resources. As a result, the placement programme was withdrawn prematurely, unilaterally and at short notice. This compromised the Crewe-based service development particularly, since they had recruited their staff later than had Birmingham. Consequently, fewer of their staff had the experience of seeing Henderson 'live', before actually going live themselves. The unilateral nature of the withdrawal also soured Henderson's relationship with Crewe, at least to an extent.

The purity of the placement experience had been sullied by the fact that some staff had been given specific (extra) tasks to undertake, at the same time. This constrained their freedom to imbibe both Henderson's structure and culture. The mix of staff in placements was not always as diverse as had been hoped, since this might have facilitated more discussion during the placement. There was relatively little informal mixing between visitors and Henderson staff, after the initial period, due to a combination of staff shortage and hosting fatigue in relation to so many 'guests' with too few recovery breaks.

The delays with recruiting, and the order in which recruitment was carried out, meant that the planned training programmes could not go ahead as originally envisaged. In particular the '5 x 2 days' training course design was produced only once, becoming corrupted into a residential crash course, which was delivered twice. The latter did not allow for gradual assimilation and discussion but probably provided more team-building, which had become a necessary aim, because of the proximity of opening and the late recruitment. Given that the courses had to be put on (i.e. staffed by Henderson and Volunteers) during the peak summer holiday period, the two residential courses went tolerably well. The atmosphere was pressurised, however, and there was much anxiety over how the new services would actually perform. This showed itself especially in relation to concern over the status of the courses – were they work or training – and the intrusion of role considerations, which emphasised the staff hierarchy, rather than its flattening, in the delegates attending. The latter two courses were not as much fun as they might have been.

Part II

The New Services in Operation

CHAPTER THREE

First Helpings

Introduction

The Steering Group overseeing the whole replication project had planned for the two new services to open approximately three months apart. This was to permit ease of visiting by HDT and also the independent organisational researcher. In the event the residential components opened only one week apart – on 12 and 19 September 2000 respectively in South Birmingham and Crewe. Consequently there was a need to reorganise the schedule of visits, and this meant that I was less present in each service than had been originally envisaged and deemed desirable. (I still had Director responsibilities to maintain at Henderson, as well as needing to preserve my sanity and some quality of life outside of work, so could not increase my input.)

This crucial phase of the service development thus found HDT, in cricketing parlance, on the back foot – reacting to events and struggling to do its job. We were struggling to address the necessary support and training needs of the new services and to find time to discuss in sufficient detail, within our team, how we thought the services were developing. Maintaining the cohesion of HDT was consequently made more difficult. Communication was poor between the HDT and the Local Implementation Teams, set up to complement our input and to prepare the service for each of our visits. So-called 'Replication Meetings', comprising HDT member, Clinical Directors and Lead Nurses from each of the three services, had been instituted (see Chapter 4). This was in order to review the progress being made, in addition to the Steering Group meetings, the agenda of which was already uncomfortably full (see Chapter 5).

Throughout this crucial period, HDT kept notes, in our collective diary, on how the visits to the new services were going. The form of recording was cryptic, because such record keeping was mainly to keep the team abreast of developments in the event of absences, of which there were relatively few. (It was never intended that they should be used for the purpose of book writing.) For the reader's ease of understanding, however, as the notes alone might be hard to decipher, the whole 'text' is provided (in italics) but with an explanatory note. The latter represents, to an extent, a measuring of the new services against the yardstick of Henderson, at least as the collective HDT viewed it – not that we were always of one mind. This chapter covers approximately the first six months of visits by HDT, the first six months' operation of the two new TCs.

The early weeks

The first few weeks post-opening were hectic. Anxiety levels were high. All struggled with surviving this period and trying to get a semblance of the Henderson programme in place. Although this was the goal, the means whereby this was to be achieved differed in the two developing services.

Overall, HDT's impression was that South Birmingham was operating an egalitarian approach with almost everything up for debate and agreement between staff and residents. By contrast, Webb House in Crewe had taken a more directive approach. In their early weeks, the latter appeared to be delivering faster progress in the direction of the Henderson's TC approach. One marker of this was the fact that the resident group appeared to consolidate more quickly, evidenced by the maintaining of higher resident numbers than in Main House in Birmingham. However, each had involved differing numbers of residents and admission at different rates, having utilised different start-up strategies. Resident numbers seemed to soar in Crewe while in Birmingham there appeared to be a ceiling effect, around the 13 mark.

None of us knew what to expect nor what the 'correct' order or speed of developmental milestones might be. Such 'not knowing' served to make us less confident and more anxious. Therefore, it was in this shared state of ignorance that we can take up the story, at the (approximately) ten weeks' stage. (N.B. Visits were equally spread between Birmingham and Crewe, but reports of some diary entries are omitted if they would have served only to make points already made.)

28 November 2000 – Crewe

Not expecting me. Community meeting with structure but without real evidence of group perspective or of team-work. However, in the second slot there was a sticking to the task that was impressive given an unexpected item and a packed agenda. The lunchtime meeting was a shambles! There had been no adequate prior discussion of purpose of session and inadequate protection in terms of attendance of relevant membership. The idea of role-play, however, was appropriate.

'NOT EXPECTING ME'

It can be seen from the above entry to the collective diary, that the apparently straightforward matter of communicating HDT visits to the new sites, via the Local Implementation Teams, was problematic. It was hard for each to hold the other in mind. In part, this probably derived from the fact that 'training' was of secondary importance – both for HDT members, who still had their 'day' jobs at

Henderson, and for new staff struggling to survive clinically but also to model themselves on another, distant service. HDT was a regular reminder of their requirement to replicate. This could serve to undermine confidence in a team that might have preferred to develop otherwise – in a direction it determined for itself.

'COMMUNITY MEETING…WITHOUT REAL EVIDENCE OF GROUP PERSPECTIVE OR OF TEAM-WORK'

When fully functioning, the Henderson model of democratic TC is represented, six mornings out of seven, by a meeting of all residents and all clinical staff on duty that day – a community meeting of around 40 people. This often feels 'large', sometimes uncomfortably so. There is no manual, nor even an accepted guiding theory, to inform staff (approximately ten of them in the meetings at any one time) as to how to perform in this setting, individually and collectively – how active to be and in what role – facilitator, teacher, (very occasionally) 'expert'. Nor is it easy to keep an awareness of one's own role and (active) contribution in relation to that of the rest of the team. As a rule of thumb, it is probably better if staff do not speak consecutively but allow residents space between, in which to respond. But then exceptions abound. Sometimes these exceptions are symbolic of some 'dynamic' that has become established between staff and residents, entered into unwittingly. Sometimes such systemic enactment needs to become a topic for discussion during the staff's after-group for unpacking and understanding, especially in relation to 'splitting'. What is also important is that the staff construe the resident group as a whole – even if the latter is not obviously functioning as a 'unit' – and also view themselves as a single system. By so construing, important inter-system aspects surface for reflection and discussion (see Main's definition of 'culture of enquiry', p.20), i.e. part of the core business of the democratic TC.

Neither the staff as a team nor the residents as a team (i.e. 'sub-systems' in their own right) was a construction that the new staff seemed to be able to perceive while actually involved in the clinical encounter, for example, in the daily community meeting. Maybe HDT was expecting too much of such new teams that they might be able to function in this way. Perhaps high levels of familiarity and trust within a team, taken for granted by those in longstanding and relatively well-functioning teams (hence ourselves), are prerequisites.

'THE LUNCHTIME MEETING WAS A SHAMBLES!'

Some aspects of this lunchtime staff meeting still stick vividly in my mind. The Henderson model requires staff to come together, Monday to Friday, in a range of lunchtime staff meetings (see Table 1.1). These include business, supervision, academic and team awareness ('sensitivity') meetings. Indirectly they act so as to promote team cohesion – at least that is one of their aims. A routine has developed that enables all staff to know in advance, at least in general terms, what the meeting is to be about. This appeared not to be the case on this occasion in Crewe, engendering uncertainty and anxiety. (Also some staff on duty were mysteriously missing from the meeting.) There was a lack of negotiation about the subject matter and the means used to explore this. The use of role-play (never utilised within the team at Henderson in the last 15 years at least) was a creative idea, but failed to deliver, in our view for want of attention to prior communication and consensus agreement. Overall this was interpreted by HDT as evidence of a team struggling to come together to work within a flattened staff hierarchy, with the need for involvement and ownership in decision-making (especially where a relatively unknown technique, with the potential to be personally exposing, was being deployed). I hope that, with HDT's feedback, this apparent 'shambles' became a source of learning to them.

29 November 2000 – Birmingham

Some evidence of structure in community meeting. Too much early focus on individuals and a lack of group thinking. Important aspects of handover left out. Staff team largely passive. The following session seemed to get some engagement with relevant issues. Powerful sense (acknowledged) of disempowerment both by staff and residents. Complaints about lack of a flattened hierarchy. NB An absence of senior staff.

'SOME EVIDENCE OF…'

The following day's visit by the 'Birmingham HDT' (i.e. different Charge Nurse, Social Therapist and Volunteers, though with me in common) revealed some similarity to that just reported. The South Birmingham team was also struggling to see the wood for the trees. It really did appear that focusing on an individual resident was an almost irresistible temptation. As discussed above, the reasons for this are not entirely clear and likely to be multiple. Within any team, but perhaps especially in a new team, there is bound to be rivalry. On this day the absence of senior staff might have created, as well as anxiety, competition over who should demonstrate leadership, and the form this could have taken might have been concentration on an individual resident. Thus, this could have been the means of communicating clinical prowess to the wider group, hence establishing dominance. Who knows? If this was the state of affairs at the start of the meeting, later on, the whole staff team appeared to have retreated into an inactive and leaderless state – perhaps fearing to develop their competitive tendencies with one another in so public a forum?

In the ensuing session with HDT there were complaints from the local staff about the absence of a flattened hierarchy within their team. HDT did not know if this was so and, if so, why. Senior staff were attending to other matters, and it can be convenient to scapegoat individuals, especially when they are not present to protest their innocence. It might be, therefore, that such a complaint was a welcome distraction from sibling rivalries, in the parents' collective absence. But it is in reality difficult for the hierarchy to be flattened if seniors are not seen to participate with more junior staff and to be regularly present. These and other conjectures filled our minds. But this theme of a non-flattened hierarchy in Birmingham was to recur.

5 December 2000 – Birmingham

Handover – no social content. Community meeting showing some added structure but no referred nor yesterday's feedback. Xmas discussed usefully but session interrupted by referred. This meeting overran by Henderson standards but was containing, justifying its length. All the after-groups were professionally performed. The afternoon's session was difficult to keep on track. There was a sense of staff wanting to merely offload. However, eventually there was a useful discussion of parallel processes around the theme of things forced upon oneself – from Chief Executive to Director to staff. Overall a sense of the Unit developing albeit coming up against the hurdle of three months without the protection of senior residents.

'HANDOVER – NO SOCIAL ETC…'

It can be seen from the diary entry that the socio-therapeutic side of the TC appeared to be under-valued. HDT's view was that this could have been due to the (different) shift pattern adopted for rota staff at Main House. Obviously the absence of any mention of 'social time' of itself is not synonymous with there being no social activity. But something is missing, in terms of the value attached to such a potentially therapeutic aspect, when no mention of it is made – either positively or negatively. Interestingly, in their subsequent community meeting, no feedback was formally invited about the previous day, given the absence of standing items relating to 'referred meetings' and 'yesterday's feedback'. These omissions therefore testified, potentially at least, to relegation in importance of 'social' or informal aspects relative to the formal programme of group activities (small psychotherapy groups, psychodrama, art therapy, work groups, etc.).

'…USEFUL DISCUSSION OF PARALLEL PROCESSES'

It was noted that the staff attending the HDT session seemed little interested in reflecting on their own functioning, deciding rather to vent their frustrations. It was as if they experienced themselves solely as hapless victims of a relentless 'top down' crushing process that paid them scant regard. Having also heard (in another forum) the seniors in this system speak of their lack of being heard by their own Trust's hierarchy (particularly in relation to the paucity of management support), it was possible to float the idea of their suffering a similar plight, albeit this was the opposite to that perceived by the 'juniors'. The notion was that there was a parallel process, operating at different levels within the TC hierarchy (that of the managers/that of the managed). At each level was experienced a similar range of beliefs and emotions – not being listened to and feeling disempowered or impotent. This phenomenon has been reported in relation to organisations, including therapeutic communities. It can be a useful tool with which to understand certain organisational difficulties. Hence apparently unfathomable and opaque problems encountered at one level within the organisation can be understood by considering happenings at a different level, which by contrast are relatively transparent and circumscribed. In relation to TC staff team dynamics and residents' sub-systems, knowing about this phenomenon of parallel process can sometimes shed useful light on what appears to be an intractable problem in one particular part of the TC. Here, it was by no means clear whether HDT's 'insight' actually was illuminating.

The hurdle of three months

It is a clinical impression at Henderson, that residents experience particular difficulties around three months into their stay. It is as if they are challenged severely to push themselves beyond this point – to delve more deeply into their problems and confront entrenched defences against change. Many do not take up the challenge posed and vote with their feet – they leave. Those who do stay beyond this point tend to stay to conclusion – between nine and twelve months. In these new services, by definition, none had witnessed this phenomenon – a transient crisis of confidence in themselves and the TC can therefore result. At Henderson, there is a familiarity and confidence based on both residents and staff having been through it all before. Even then there are dropouts from treatment, and staff are not emotionally unaffected by this. HDT therefore soon realised that we were witnessing a particularly painful part of the process of setting up, as the whole system seemed to become acutely depressed and demoralised. Christmas was also coming and both units were to remain in the grip of this despair for some time.

6 December 2000 – Crewe

Handover lacked an adequate sense of boundary. There was too much inattention, coffee-making etc. The community meeting did show more structuring than previously but although promised, there was no yesterday's feedback. This passed without staff comment. The review was also rather an un-boundaried affair. The next session with staff centred on individual cases i.e. residents. There was much anxiety especially concerning the physical health of residents. It was difficult to facilitate the group to think, in terms of the TC model about such examples and a number of staff present (mainly junior) felt insufficiently supervised. Difficult to know how much 'splitting' we might be caught in.

NB The previous evening had been marked by one-to-ones with the volunteers being caught up in some in-house situations.

NNB Both services seemed to be facing similar 3-months phenomena, well-known to Henderson, but potentially undermining since neither residents nor staff have experience of going beyond this point nor of success – a difficult hurdle to cross.

NNNB Idea of Xmas at Crewe introduced – might need reiteration.

'HANDOVER LACKED…'

Handover in the morning, to which this diary entry refers, is a crucial time. It is a meeting between a bleary-eyed minority (night staff) and the bushy-tailed majority (day staff), with often much to report and little time to interact. Performance anxieties can run high not only about the work undertaken during the previous night shift but also about how coherently it is presented to the rest of the team present. Even weather-beaten, battle-hardened Henderson staff struggle to do this handover function justice. What is encountered between the two tired 'performers' taking centre stage, is also the way in which they cooperate, complement or contradict one another. Variations of this often weary interaction also indirectly, and non-verbally, communicate something of the reality of the previous 16 hours of TC life.

Given the above, which obtains when the TC system is working optimally, HDT took it to be relevant that there was noticeable 'inattention' during handover. Now, not all staff actually do arrive bright-eyed and bushy-tailed – some are by nature more night owls than larks! In the main, however, such idiosyncrasies tend to be absent or else masked, and generally there exists a high level of respect for those handing over (and for the process itself), which disallows the making of coffee or indeed any other activity at this crucial time of the day. So this was a noteworthy departure from the Henderson handover procedure.

What was the 'something' that all this might mean? The later mention of the review of the community meeting being also 'rather an un-boundaried affair' gives a clue. There had been difficulty with identifying the discrete 'structural' elements of the programme – the different meetings – as fulfilling particular functions. So it was as if handover was also a kind of pre-match limbering up before appearing on the field of play with the residents, rather than what it should have been – namely, part of the match itself. (N.B. At Webb House in Crewe the two night staff met before the official handover to present their findings to their Lead Nurse. This method, which deviated from the process at Henderson, was instituted intentionally (but unilaterally) by the new staff team in order to support those handing over, in recognition of the difficulty and importance of the task – their Lead Nurse was an ex-Henderson Charge Nurse. Paradoxically, this well-intentioned departure may have served to relegate the handover proper in its importance.)

Like Main House, Webb was struggling with getting a handle on the residents, as a group, and not just as a collection of individuals. This was revealed in the second session's meeting with HDT. It was noted that physical ill health was a preoccupation with the staff. To an extent, the concern over physical illness (not in itself inappropriate) acted so as to draw back many staff into their former, clearer and more comfortable roles – doctors and nurses. (In fact, Webb had never intended to replicate Henderson's 'surgery' function. They viewed it as pretentious that we called it a 'surgery', when there was no qualified family doctor present to oversee it. As a result a trainee GP had been hired by them, though having little prior psychiatric experience.)

At least at this point, in Crewe, what HDT witnessed appeared to be a retreat into safe medical territory in the face of psychological bewilderment and worry regarding an eating-disordered resident. It was hard for new staff to stand back from the concreteness of the physical implications of the individual resident's disorder and to see themselves as staff in relation to a person presenting with serious symptoms – in both mind and body. It was as if these two aspects had been dislocated from one another. This resident therefore was not in fact receiving a holistic treatment, and psychiatric staff were denying something of the reality of their own profession in discussing only the somatic aspects.

The response to HDT's comments in this session was for the staff present to blame their seniors for providing too little supervision and also indirectly to criticise HDT for not having trained them better! This represented another instance of potential 'splitting', between senior/junior or (clinical) managers/managed. HDT thus felt itself to be at one apex of a triangle at both new service sites – with 'seniors' and 'juniors' at the other two apices. Many factors contributed to this. Rivalry and competition amongst the three Directors should also be entertained as a possible factor. It was tempting for HDT (including Henderson's Director – me) to side with the juniors as under-supported and under-supervised, while experiencing ourselves as their rescuers from sub-standard local senior staff – actually our peers and close professional collaborators.

14 December 2000 – Crewe

Overnight to Crewe, involving volunteers. Only KN attended the community meeting. Previous had been difficult with one staff member bearing the brunt. The result was a divided community – staff and residents. Agreed for volunteers to meet residents during second slot while HDT staff met Crewe staff. After lunch all HDT members met staff alone. Looked at ways of understanding and resolving the split – hopefully a useful meeting.

There are difficulties with stand alone posts e.g. social worker, art therapist etc. Perhaps some cross-site linkages could be established? Boundaries remained a problem with a lack of clarity about referred meetings – membership and timing. Important to recognise the role of a clear structure and how this can be therapeutic and more important than simply being kind. Handovers also need to be clear in terms of membership, timing and place.

The only comment to add here is in regard to the boundary issue – to underline the importance of it. What did not seem to be understood by the new Crewe team was the rationale for aspects of the programme, for example, that for involving all staff on duty in attending a referred meeting. Having all staff present maximises communication between staff and provides emotional containment for residents through their experiencing the continuity of staff presence. The 'splits' identified by HDT could be worsened by having some staff in and other staff out of such meetings. The full significance of handover still seemed to be misunderstood.

2 January 2001 – Crewe

Missed the community meeting but caught the after-group. A good discussion and seemingly an appropriately negative backlash against staff in this meeting, following a relatively intimate Christmas period. The after-group got started very promptly which contrasted with before Christmas. One of the staff (charge nurse) has a plan to document the procedures for 'nights', partly to help improve consistency and partly to document changes and developments with time. Only one resident had left over Christmas. The Director was on leave, although KN had spoken between Christmas and the New Year. Lead nurse wondered if the 'original residents' in Birmingham, as at Crewe, were undermining the formal Top 3 structure – an interesting hypothesis. Still issues around seeing the residents as a group, to avoid an undue focus on a given individual, while recognising the paradox that the actual cohesion of residents is more apparent than real. The residents still give rise to a lot of expression of negative counter-transference, which is essentially un-challenged and un-explored – probably within normal limits and serving a cathartic function and helping with team cohesion! Morale seemed high.

'…NEGATIVE BACKLASH AGAINST STAFF'

This observed post-Christmas phenomenon is typical and also interesting. What we have repeatedly found at Henderson is that the shrinking of the resident numbers (and also staff numbers) over the Christmas period, as those who have places to go leave for the festive period, often creates a level of intimacy (or at least of shared experiences and the appearance of intimacy) in those remaining that does not ordinarily obtain. This means that as the full TC resumes there is a problem with re-integrating those who were absent. Feelings of envy and destructive responses arising out of this may surface in relation to those who did have 'places to go' – often envisaged as glorious havens of peace and tranquillity. But this difficulty – negative backlash – is better, in psychological health terms, than a flat denial of difficulties or a sulking retreat. (N.B. The re-integration process involves both staff and residents.)

'ORIGINAL RESIDENTS...UNDERMINING...'

Having got through the troublesome three months' stage, it may be that these residents from the first cohort to have been admitted gained in confidence. However, what they faced next was that those residents who had arrived in later cohorts were now eligible to take up the lead resident roles – namely 'Top Three'. If the observation about undermining was accurate then, presumably, there were feelings of rivalry and maybe envy. These therefore lay behind any 'undermining', although part of this competition might also represent a healthy competitive struggle. The level of difficulty posed by this situation was again related to the fact that this new service was encountering this phenomenon, as with so many others, for the first time. In an established TC, such as Henderson, it is common-place to see existing Top Three residents and seniors coming into confrontation, and not uncommon for the newer Top Three to bow to their seniors' superior knowledge and wisdom, though not always gracefully. (Being sometimes in a formal leadership role and sometimes on the receiving end of it may itself be an important part of the democratic TC experience, part of what is therapeutic.) Transitions, into and out of posts of relative power, reveal those who require the protection of a role in order to perform effectively and those who do not. Some residents only have a 'voice' when in a formal role. Such matters form the subject of psychotherapeutic exploration within the formal programme of group meetings (see Whiteley 1986).

'A LOT OF EXPRESSION OF NEGATIVE COUNTER-TRANSFERENCE'

An amount of indirectly and directly expressed negativity towards residents from staff had gone unchallenged. The full reasons for this were not understood by HDT. Inevitably there are frustrations, especially during the course of this type of clinical work, and additionally so when it is part of an innovative enterprise, as with the replication project. One function of 'after-groups' is to allow ventilation of negative feelings, which can provide a relief to staff members and also allow for differences of opinion to be safely expressed. Importantly, however, such ventilation needs to prompt questions of just what is going on within the TC – part of the necessary 'culture of enquiry' (see Main 1983). It is not unusual for some staff to feel 'positive' while others feel 'negative' in relation to the same event, issue or person. Provided all reactions are expressed freely, the scene is set for healthy discussion and potentially in-depth understanding (see Norton 1997b).

At Henderson, discussion and understanding, if not available at the after-group, would be sought for in the weekly supervision and/or team awareness meetings. In order to maximise the therapeutic potential of the inpatient environment, it is important that staffs' counter-transference reactions should be sustained rather than suppressed (Gabbard 1986). Only then can these be examined (within the democratic TC model, in a range of group settings as above) so that any unconscious communication from residents might be gleaned. It is one of the tasks of clinical leaders within the TC to try to strike the right balance between permitting a healthy catharsis of negative (or indeed positive) feeling towards residents and introducing the scrutiny of such aspects. To an extent, catharsis can help with staff team cohesion. However, beyond a certain point, which is difficult to define with any certainty, the expression of negativity towards residents tends to represent the effects of powerful splitting influences. (Positive aspects are displaced thereby, often on to some subgroup of the staff team.) Chronically unchallenged, these negative 'projections' may lead to a serious breakdown in collaboration between the two most important sub-systems within the democratic TC – staff and residents – and dangerous acting out can be fostered.

As is noted, HDT's report here concluded that what had been witnessed was 'probably within normal [i.e. Henderson] limits'. (HDT may not therefore have brought up this matter for further discussion.) The fact that only one resident had failed to return following the Christmas break could have given the staff team reason for confidence in their capacity to provide for the therapeutic needs of their residents, hence morale could be high. Alternatively, this might have been due to the fact that all negativity had been displaced into the residents, thereby allowing the staff team to feel positive about itself. It can be seen from these comments that HDT had to judge when to confront and intervene with the new teams and when not. Too much intervention, and we might demoralise, undermining confidence or inducting a defensive passivity and dependence on us. Too little intervention, and we could tacitly reinforce inappropriate attitudes and behaviour. Encountering so many novel stages and phenomena, the new staff teams were at times easily feeling criticised or attacked. HDT, staff and Volunteers, usually felt constrained in what they could express of a negative kind, perhaps overly so. Volunteers tended to be freer in their criticism (or at least more direct than HDT staff) and better heard than HDT staff when they raised concerns, although some new staff also felt criticised by them.

3 January 2001 – Birmingham

Arrived mid-morning and spent some informal time with staff. All twelve residents had returned following Christmas. Supervision session was very impressive with an in-depth discussion of relevant dynamic and systemic issues. Interestingly there was a wish for the volunteers to begin the phased withdrawal from the project. Their input had been highly valued and it was felt that they still had much to offer discharge groups and in relation to the whole leaving process. Their absence might make it clearer what role the current residents might fulfil. (NB: This came out of a session taking place after the supervision.)

In Birmingham therefore there was a similar feeling of post-Christmas break success, in that all 12 of their residents had returned. It is not clear therefore if 'confidence' was reflected in a wish to do away with dependency on HDT – at least the Volunteer aspect of this. Some of the more outspoken criticism from Volunteers, referred to above, might also have contributed. However, what was enacted here, perhaps, was some form of collusion between HDT staff and Main House staff, since the discussion about withdrawing Volunteers had occurred when the Volunteers had not been present. Ordinarily, as HDT, we would have discussed this suggestion with Volunteers, especially if they had not been party to it. It may have been some form of splitting therefore within our team that was being enacted. (N.B. Supervision of our HDT staff function had been mooted around December 2000, so as to enable us to maintain our objectivity, through ventilating feelings and acknowledging differences of opinions.) As staff in the HDT, we had agreed that current residents might in future have a role to play – functionally replacing the Volunteers. At our next meeting with the latter, however, they made it clear to us that this was a bad idea, principally because unlike themselves, current Henderson residents had not experienced leaving (and its aftermath) and so were ill-placed to advise on this crucial stage of the therapeutic process. The timing for such a change of HDT personnel was consequently all wrong. Somewhat with our tails between our legs, HDT staff re-negotiated with Main House staff the continuation of the role of Volunteers for the eminently sensible reasons articulated by the latter.

The reference to 'current residents' referred to the original plan to involve current as well as ex-residents in detecting the authentic aroma of a replicated Henderson service. In this respect, it might be argued that current rather than ex-residents should have the keener noses. The idea was that the new services would resemble the 'modern' Henderson, not a (relatively) antique rendition recalled by ex-residents. This idea was not in fact realised, and only much later (over a year post-opening) was there any cross-flow of current residents among the three services (and that with difficulty and only once). Up to this point, the role of the current services had been largely limited to that of advising on the selection of the new premises and the refurbishment – not unimportant aspects of the project.

Birmingham entry dated 30 January 2001

Previous week – no notes but a shambolic '9.30' (community meeting) with 29 items announced by Chair and only three achieved by Community but without any apparent concern, judging by after-group. 'Res Reps' (equivalent to Henderson's 'Top Three') were relatively junior and undermined by senior residents and staff who were also undermining one another, having gone on to the meeting unprepared/unresolved with respect to 'reviews' issue.

No sense of urgency/prioritising so unclear what next session was to be and 'reviews' were to go ahead without any reviewee(!) – though in the event one review did take place.

Staff and volunteers arrived late, 12 noon, due to continuing major rail problems, thus together we faced a 2½ hour lunch break – organisation of HDT interface needs overhaul!

Following HDT meeting decided to propose 'after-group' to examine feelings, not least because of 'resistance' noted at recent HDT meeting in Sutton and KN's negative feelings from the morning. That bit was productive with Birmingham's staff ambivalent feelings to HDT being acknowledged. Negotiation needed.

'A SHAMBOLIC "9.30" (COMMUNITY MEETING)'

At this memorable meeting, the resident Chair had announced that there were to be 29 items on the agenda that morning – no regular or standing items having become part of the structure of this meeting, which at Henderson is highly organised (see Chapter 1). The striking fact here was the acceptance of this state of affairs, which meant that almost certainly the vast majority of items would not be covered or, if so, only very inadequately. Bearing in mind that with the Henderson model it is the 'process' more than the 'product' that is of the essence, the accent is on the quality not quantity of the community's work. This is seen nowhere more clearly than in the community meeting, although there is always a balance to be struck between the process and product. In this instance, it was never likely that 20-plus items could be adequately presented, discussed and agreed with a meeting lasting but 60 minutes – Birmingham had not modelled Henderson's 75-minute meeting!

Neither residents nor staff appeared concerned that the quality and amount of business were pitted against one another within such an agenda. And, to make matters worse, each party seemed intent on undermining itself. There was little sense of cohesion between the two main sub-systems – staff and residents. Regarding the latter, the senior residents tended to cling to the power vested in them by virtue of being longer within the treatment, in spite of formally having relinquished their status in favour of newer residents i.e. those who had assumed the 'Top Three' (in this case 'Res Rep') posts. It may not be a coincidence that Birmingham's non-acceptance of the term 'Top Three' was associated with a (relative) disempowerment by those who were merely 'representatives' and not 'on top'.

The absence of concern about the size of the agenda meant that there was no prioritising of items, and it remained unclear, in the face of so much work left unattended to, what the morning's second session in the programme was to be. This state of affairs at Henderson Hospital would be almost unthinkable, since there is usually a strong desire for a predictable environment. The disorganisation continued into the next session of the day's programme, with the planned three months' review of residents' progress, but without the residents being informed so as to be able to prepare themselves adequately. Such a chaotic situation might represent a recapitulation of their childhood when as children they were moved more as commodities than sentient beings. For a three months' review, the resident sub-system has to report progress (in terms of attendance in groups, groups missed, jobs held, rules transgressed, etc. within the previous three months in the community). This also requires prior notification. Remarkably, some structure did emerge from these unpromising beginnings in the form of a single resident being reviewed in the session before lunch. Henderson would have reviewed three in the same time. But this was not Henderson – at least not yet.

More shambles had ensued courtesy of Virgin Trains, meaning that the rest of HDT (i.e. not me – I had left the train behind, choosing to drive myself to and between venues) arrived just in time for the lunch break! On this occasion, in the absence of arrangements being made for us during the lunch period, the break lasted two and a half hours. This was a desperate situation captured in the diary by characteristic understatement – 'HDT interface needs overhaul' (i.e. interface between HDT and the Local Implementation Team). HDT, staff and residents were fuming, largely in the direction of Richard Branson (head of Virgin Trains) but partly at our professional colleagues from Main House. HDT had adopted a kind of 'after-group' within the group this week, with staff from the new service in Birmingham, so as to process the training session. We had noted that staff had often seemed unfulfilled, and providing space for such views to be explored found local favour. Birmingham staff could now acknowledge ambivalence more openly.

30 January 2001 – Birmingham

This week – more of a sense of HDT being expected, welcomed and wanted. Reminder by Henderson sent the day before. Handover left staff unprepared? Because of lack of leaders (no Clinical Director or Lead Nurse), left to 'middle management' and others – especially the six residents to selection pronouncement from Outreach/Managers. Sense of insufficient decisions being made in the community, both whole staff team meetings and (9.30). Splitting evident.

Community meeting – only two residents – typical of obstacles posed by small numbers and excessive staff, leading to lack of face valid evidence of empowerment of residents, when in such a minority.

Buffet lunch (brilliant idea) but ? whole community because of still 'us and them' as observed by A (Charge nurse) last week.

Henderson Lead Nurses' presence – welcomed – what have we been missing? Still she may be able to make fortnightly from next week on Wednesdays.

Afternoon slot 2.30–3.30 caught up in split, in spite of knowing and talking about this. 'Keeping up appearances' when HDT present and ?Lead Nurse and Clinical Director keeping up appearances as happy couple, as defence?

Suggestion that we have communal lunch next time and shift ownership of programme towards local service? They are building antipathy to volunteers (??HDT staff).

Perhaps there was less ambivalence around, as it turned out that the HDT had been expected – more than that, 'welcomed and wanted'. What a pity we had not thought to introduce after-groups into our previous sessions. On that day, however, staff did not appear ready for their clinical task in the absence of usual senior staff. The previous day's 'selection meeting' had been heavy, with six candidates being interviewed (Henderson Hospital's maximum is four), and there was a sense of disempowerment, in that the Outreach limb of the service had dictated that so many candidates should be interviewed. Decisions were felt by residential staff in the new service to be made in forums of which they were not a part. Consequently, there was a strong feeling of 'them and us' within their clinical team.

The whole empowerment edifice seemed to have crumbled, even before it solidly existed, with a vast excess of staff in the community meeting relative to residents. The residents felt disempowered but then the staff present with them also felt similarly (see p.000 for discussion of 'parallel processes'). A buffet lunch had been arranged but this failed to bring the whole community together as planned. The Nurse Manager from Henderson (Lyn Suddards) had joined the HDT on that particular visit and appeared (to us) as a breath of fresh air. In spite of this, we felt caught up in the 'them and us', believing that the senior staff felt they had to keep up appearances in front of their own staff, in spite of private feelings that everything in the garden might not be so rosy. It was acknowledged that the communal lunch might still be a good idea, and would bring together warring factions.

HDT felt that the Local Implementation Team should take more responsibility for the training sessions, ensuring that local staff would be available and determining what they wanted to discuss. At the same time, HDT (at least its staff) were sensing that there was a growing South Birmingham antipathy towards the Volunteer voices of the HDT. All in all there was a great sense of fragmentation and not a little ill feeling, not much of which seemed to be able to be talked about openly and directly. Throwing food at the problem (via the communal lunch) seemed to be the best that any of us could think to do to improve matters.

31 January 2001 – Crewe

Overnight with staff and volunteers (although one volunteer had to leave early the following morning before communal breakfast). KN late for 7.45 am meeting – thought 8 am breakfast. Notes taken of breakfast meeting – more logic/chronology to handover; currently less individual-centred but ? facilitated by Volunteers more than by Crewe staff.

Good, authentic feel to 9.30 except insufficient attention to previous day and to relatively inactive residents, i.e. not reported in referred meetings.

Useful meeting with staff re feeding back re previous night's business – though the weakness of HDT model is the absence of actual participating staff in the session.

Drug error reported –? Counter-transference reaction suggested by KN to introduce pychodynamic thinking.

Discussed future agenda in terms of problem scenarios and how HDT to spend time with residents if not in overnight format.

As was becoming usual practice, after my visit to Birmingham I travelled to Crewe in the evening, to meet up with that part of HDT which had been visiting Webb House there during the day and the evening. In practice, this meant catching up with the rest of the Crewe team at breakfast the next morning, since the visit lasted till after the evening's summit meeting between duty staff and residents i.e. 10.30 p.m. These evening visits to the social part of the programme (carried out by Volunteers, nursing staff and Social Therapists, i.e. those that knew what went on – not me) were felt by the local services to be very helpful and also revealing in terms of what went on during the informal time of the programme.

The following morning I was late for breakfast, thinking that it was an eight o'clock start, whereas it was 7.45 a.m.! The previous evening's handover had been observed to improve with evidence of a chronological account of the day that encompassed more relevant business hence a shade 'more logic'. It was noted that it was less individually centred, although it was not clear whether the Volunteers had somehow engineered this rather than its having emanated from the new staff themselves.

After breakfast, that morning's community meeting felt 'authentic', although for HDT's taste there was too little emphasis in it on what had happened during the previous day. Residents were relatively inactive. The meeting with staff that followed was seen to be useful, the topic being the feeding in of the previous evening's/night's business. However, discussion about how to hand over adequately probably would not have reached the ears of those who worked the previous night – a severe limitation of the HDT practice that would prove impossible to resolve fully. We had to assume that what we witnessed on a given day applied at all times and to all staff, although we knew this was not likely to be the case.

Interestingly, on this visit, an error in prescribing/dispensing of medication had occurred. This provided HDT with an opportunity not only to observe how the new staff dealt with this administratively but also to examine with them how psychodynamic factors between residents and staff might also impact on the apparently straightforward 'medical' transaction – medication. HDT tended to be adaptable and to seize training opportunities, such as this event posed, rather than to arrive with a pre-ordained agenda. Having said that, what followed in this visit was a new plan for the local service to identify 'problem scenarios' that then could be discussed with HDT subsequently when we visited. One such was how to deal with a resident who was discharged by TC in the middle of the night, i.e. without the complete range of health and social resource available.

Change of plans

Because of continuing train delays it was proposed that instead of the one day per week visiting format, Tuesdays in Birmingham, Wednesdays in Crewe (or vice-versa), HDT would spend two days per fortnight in each service. Day 1 of the two would be substantially as it had been up till then, and as reported, but without working during the evening. Day 2 would include the following day's programme up until the lunchtime meeting, after which the team would return to London. In practice, this meant meeting at Euston Station somewhere between 7.00 and 7.30 a.m. on a Tuesday and returning there late Wednesday afternoon. (For rota staffing purposes this was formulated as equivalent to working two 10-hour days – the total time spent away from home was nearer 36 hours.)

For me this new plan brought a more relaxed schedule, since I did not have to straddle both sites each week and could therefore feel a more settled part of the HDT, even though I continued to travel separately, since the trains remained so unreliable and since I felt my duty lay in 'being there' for the new services – the road was more reliable than the rail! The result was some ongoing fragmentation within the HDT and a greater reliance upon its rota staff members. However, the evening meal format, spent with staff and Volunteers together in the hotel restaurant, seemed to heal most of the rifts as far as we could tell. So, fortnightly meetings would continue till the end of the first six months' period, i.e. until mid-March 2001. Thereafter, given the continuing train problems, there would be six months of the new two-day blocks format, monthly rather than the scheduled fortnightly visits. We could not anticipate what might result from such departures from the original plan.

6/7 February 2001 –Birmingham

The last visit had apparently been satisfactory according to both K and J. However the numbers of residents remained low as did staff morale. Clearly there are many factors operating including X's leaving, the low numbers, the early stage of the development, the previous day's staff absence due to a scheduled meeting and the previous day/evening's difficulty. The Wednesday saw no senior staff (above H grade) and some uncertainty about duty staff, i.e. whether a nurse was essential or not. My question about who would lead any 'fire-related situation' was met with bemusement. Later I was approached by a member of the team to give advice concerning the ongoing management of the crisis from a previous day.

From the formal sessions, there were initially no staff available, having to reschedule the timing, who were able to discuss what had been agreed – mainly small and large groups. We developed this theme to look also at the staff split and the accompanying sense of disempowerment, which was felt in much of the Unit.

We had arranged in the community meeting to meet with residents at lunchtime and stressed the need to identify the positives and also to structure the community meeting via the agenda – something also covered in the am meeting and covered many times before. This time the slot was on representing a 'bridge' between the small and the large group.

The final session with staff centred on the staff split and how unheard the more junior staff felt in relation to the 'managers'. We tried to explore this in terms of the parallel processes and to consider that the 'managers' might also be caught up in the same systemic process within the wider trust in the NHS.

This report reveals something of the complexity of the replication task and also the difficulty that confronted HDT at each visit. It was never entirely clear what was going on or, if there seemed to be a main issue, to what this might be attributed. On this occasion the ongoing low morale was commented upon. It seemed to reflect the incapacity of the Unit to contain its residents – to retain them in treatment – and to build to a number that would allow fuller community participation. Were this building up of numbers to happen, a greater sense of empowerment might develop. Without this, the low numbers would inevitably mean that residents were often in the minority and thus, in spite of the staff protest to the opposite, the residents' feeling of actual empowerment would be almost impossible to engender.

The fact that one of the more senior and apparently enthusiastic staff was leaving only added to the sense of low morale. The reasons surrounding this move were unclear to HDT, although theories about the leaving were legion. To the junior staff it appeared that this member had in some way stepped out of line or fallen from favour with managerial colleagues. Therefore they represented something of a heroic figure, if not a martyr. It was not clear, however, what was the just cause with which this human casualty might be aligned. The recent senior staff absence was possibly connected to the leaving and probably connected to the difficulty referred to from the previous day. The fact that there were so few senior staff on duty on the particular day of the visit only added to the difficulty of the clinical task that faced them. Perhaps it was no surprise therefore that the staff present would be clutching at straws, such as asking a member of HDT, in effect, to lead the clinical team – an invitation which was declined.

The fact that the community meeting's agenda still lacked the structure as at Henderson remained a cause for concern. This occurred in spite of the relevant (written) information being disseminated on more that one occasion. One standing item on Henderson's agenda represents feedback into the community meeting of the smaller group meetings from the previous day. This item thus acts so as to integrate relevant emotional and interpersonal information from one part of the programme to another, the purpose being to integrate it or make sense of contradictions or points of confusion. HDT thus tried to unpack some of the structural elements, through introducing an underpinning rationale, with the aim of making the embedding of such structure easier.

13 February 2001 – Birmingham

Difficult backdrop with X's leaving and apparent staff splits (and HDT splits and organisational researcher splits).

The previous day had seen a SWOT (strengths, weaknesses, opportunities and threats) analysis and signs of this were littered/displayed on the walls.

An item in the 9.30 meeting about clearing up from yesterday – perhaps on the basis that 'no mess' was feasible or even desirable.

At prior handover, little social content but some sexualised 'two or one' etc material left undiscussed – ? Awkwardness avoid issue/my being present/staff split etc. (My preoccupation that decrease in social time for shift system non-replication was/is problematic.)

Sense of high profile of Outreach/senior staff not in the know who nevertheless assume responsibility/seniority or are uncomfortable with its lack. This revealed but not really explored in the review of community meeting.

Pre-lunch slot initially staff member then 2–3 concentrating on basic – 'who set out room/chairs etc' why – need for transparency 'culture of enquiry'.

Seems to be a greater freedom to ask about Henderson. My talk of stages during after-group.

The atmosphere in the Unit continued to be difficult following X's leaving as noted above. This event was intimately linked in the minds of many staff (if not also residents) with difficulties between senior and junior staff. HDT were divided on how best to respond and whether the situation was so problematic as to require some formal intervention via a communication from HDT to the higher echelons of the South Birmingham Trust. Some felt that concerns were sufficiently serious to warrant contact being made with the Clinical Director prior to the next meeting. Others felt that the situation was not so worrying – that it could wait until the next Replication Meeting. (The organisational researcher is also mentioned in this note as having become apparently affected by the issue i.e. having a professional concern about the limits of her own role and whether there might be an indication for this boundary to be transgressed through registering a concern to the Trust(s) involved. She was observing us but we were also observing her.)

It was difficult to know whether the Birmingham team's evaluation of itself, according to its strengths, weaknesses, opportunities and threats (SWOT), was a sign of optimism or its opposite. Cynically, it might be said that such an analysis was a statement of desperation. To HDT, the preoccupation with physical mess served as a distraction from the much more relevant and concerning mess that was the staff team 'dynamics' at this point. One worrying aspect of this mess was the fact (according to some junior residential staff) that there were senior clinical staff, for example Outreach staff, who took charge in community meetings, without being fully aware of current community business. It was as if they felt too uncomfortable to acknowledge ignorance in front of, or yield their status to, their junior colleagues.

The pre-lunch session with staff, albeit very thinly attended, focused on the basic structuring of the community meeting's agenda. At Henderson the community meeting starts with a question, 'Who's missing?' This is to ascertain that those missing are at least identified and possibly also accounted for. We tried to introduce a discussion of this and other practical measures, such as who sets out rooms – positions chairs, provides tissues – prior to groups. Such aspects might convey a sense of containment or welcome. Essentially we were trying to promote an understanding of why such activities might be undertaken. We tried to stress the need for transparency, in the sense of open communication between subgroups within the TC, and to establish a culture of enquiry – questioning why things were the way they were.

That day we formed the view that there was a greater sense of freedom, perhaps deriving from a lower level of anxiety, among the staff to challenge 'Henderson'. This was possibly related to our sensitivity to the fact that we did not know exactly what to expect of the community in its under-developed state – or precisely what stage it was at – but recognised that it was on a trajectory or 'learning curve'. This statement seemed to help to allow staff to voice their ignorance and to question HDT and the Henderson TC model.

28 February 2001 – Birmingham

Concerns expressed by KN to Steering group meeting two weeks ago regarding Birmingham situation since when on annual leave. KN had prior meeting with South West London St George's Trust's Clinical Director who attended subsequent meeting. Approaching 'worst case' scenario of a service deviating, in this case, in shift pattern, and potentially significantly and being out of reach of HDT intervention. At this stage, however, concern seems to be appropriately shared by Clinical Director and Lead Nurse and no further action beyond minutes etc for circulation to take place.

Visit by HDT (including KP and JR) apparently went well last week although resident numbers are still low, at 13.

Following my talk with Trust 'clinical' director I have sent apologies for yesterday and today since I felt the need to cancel my input to HDT visit to Crewe, following staff group discussion.

It is clear from the above note that the concern regarding the Birmingham situation was great. The staff team was in serious disarray, most prominently regarding the difficulties between managers and those managed. The matter was obviously discussed at the Steering Group (see Chapter 5). It was of concern to all three Trusts; hence relevant personnel were made aware of this, and not just those in Birmingham. From the outset successful replication meant that the two new services had each to replicate and that future funding *for all three* was dependent upon such a positive outcome. The failure of any single service during the process threatened the whole replication project and in particular the likelihood of subsequent funding.

At this point, what was most feared by HDT was the nightmare scenario that one of the new services would have deviated so far from the Henderson model as to make it difficult to rescue it. This situation appeared to be fast approaching. The collective diary entry is also noteworthy for my record of contacting my own Trust to alert my immediate (medical) superior to the situation, so that the relevant information was conveyed upwards to the most senior staff within our Trust. What is also clear, which would have added to my sense of anxiety at that time, was a concerning situation back at Henderson. This also needed my attention in the absence of other senior staff. This situation therefore represents an example of the chronic tension experienced by HDT staff in straddling both the development project and ordinary clinical work. This tension meant that HDT members frequently did not feel a sense of freedom to go out to the new services. Our minds were often drawn back to what was going on at Henderson.

14 March 2001 – Crewe

KN present on day one only (with JR, MB, LS and one volunteer).

Structure of the day was delivered by residents – ? breakdown in HDT / Local Implementation Team function or super-efficient? Largely resident contact Day 1 and staff contact Day 2.

Welcome went well but not able to attend review. Elections enabling Outreach to see development – beneficial – with some challenge and nominating of others. Not quite seeing 'wood for trees' in the importance of electing new Top Three – ? due to mobile small group syndrome.

Lunch with residents allowing useful informal time and the witnessing of senior (Crewe) residents teaching 'more junior residents'.

Lunchtime meeting with staff alone not well prepared, with a superficial covering of a number of topics. Only small number of staff in on the day and not all of those were present. 'Couples' developing? Unchallenged because of TC not having seen sufficient destructive effect of such couplings – up till now. (NB Missed out on informal 'after-groups' with team, during the period I was travelling exclusively by car.)

PM meeting with three residents (two new and one old) had some difficulty with containing anxiety of the two new and differentiating its HDT task from that of therapy. (Importance of volunteers cannot be underestimated – Volunteer's summary of the similarity between eating / drugs / obsessive disorder as avoidance of 'feelings' was remarkable and ? need to stop behaviour in order to feel – very pithy and persuasive!!)

Then tea and after-group – x 3 with residents, Crewe staff and HDT alone.

Good structure – important to have had a 9–5 Crewe member in PM who could represent / correct at the next day's 9.30 and after-group with HDT – triangulation.

Convivial meal and meeting with Charge Nurse. Pity that Lead Nurse unable to attend Replication [Meeting] due to low staffing – 'Replication' of low numbers.

On the one hand, in being welcomed and expected by residents in Crewe, we seemed to have overcome, at least in part, communication difficulties between HDT and the Local Implementation Team. However, we were unsure if the predominance of residents in our reception represented a resident take-over, with the staff somehow sidelined in the process. We were therefore bemused at the direct lead in greeting us being taken by residents. There was one particular resident who regularly met us and would always comment that she was about to leave the community – on that very day. In fact for a number of months this gloomy prophesy – delivered with some relish – was not realised. Such ambivalence about staying seemed to resonate with the wider ambivalence in the new staff about HDT's presence (and perhaps also some ambivalence in HDT).

'Mobile small group syndrome' is a phenomenon that is well known at Henderson. It refers to the ease with which the proper liaison function of the 'Top Three' residents shifts into one of providing support and/or therapy to those who consult this structural element. This was an interesting development, not least since it has potentially therapeutic value. Many residents struggle to be appropriately involved in others' affairs and to create a reasonable healthy distance between themselves and others. They thus habitually over- or under-invest emotionally. Taking on one of the 'Top Three' positions therefore exposes them to what in effect is a difficult balancing act. They are invited to hear of others' difficulties but have a duty to maintain a distance – to attempt to be objective and rational – and if judged necessary, to involve the whole community's resource, i.e. not just their own. Frequently, they struggle to master this interface, and often they are only partially successful in doing so. One result, as referred to here, is that the 'Top Three' together oversteps the mark and moves from merely liaising (between staff and the resident sub-systems) to providing support and therapy, hence the 'mobile small group'. This aspect was thus simultaneously replicating Henderson and also providing a learning point for all concerned.

It was gratifying to witness at lunch the fact that, true to the original Maxwell Jones observation, senior residents could be seen to be leading those more junior to them. In this instance it was regarding the transmission of the Unit's timetable and the nature of this new service development, in short the purpose for which HDT visited. The informal lunches provided a useful mechanism for Crewe residents to get to know Henderson staff and Volunteers better. Therefore they probably also contributed to an increasing ease with our being around, which might have led to our witnessing more of what the place was usually like, i.e. for us to have had less of a distorting influence over what we were observing.

At the lunchtime meeting with staff we learnt that there were 'couples' within the resident group. HDT felt that these were insufficiently challenged. The reason for this, we imagined, was the community, in being new, had not seen the destructive effect of such couplings, at least until this point. Within the context of the TC, it is easy for staff to condone relationships which superficially appear healthy. This is to deny, however, the unusual nature of the therapeutic environment – its great capacity to provide support – and its influence in masking the 'true' nature of relationships. The idea is that the new relationships encountered are in an important way experimental, yielding opportunities to compare and contrast with past relationships. When the 'as if' quality is lacking or lost, a not infrequent occurrence, intimate relationships can form that become apparently robust and stable. However, such couples cannot really know with whom they are in a relationship and can easily become falsely optimistic, believing that they are in a much better quality of relationship than is the case. This is a particularly tempting conclusion to reach when past relationships have been poor or destructive. This optimism can frequently affect not only those coupled but also other residents (and staff) as appeared to be the case here.

20/21 March 2001 – Birmingham

Morning slot – community project? Housekeeping – attended by volunteer and KN. Interesting to see that administrator led the meeting with issues mainly addressed through her – a different feel from the 'GLO' at Henderson, at least in the past where it was mainly clinical staff led therefore more liable to be therapeutic. Informal lunch with staff and meeting with 3 residents. Looking at breaking vicious circle of negativity by recognising positives and issue of drawing a line between junior and senior residents.

Handover – Looked like there would be no staff to meet with HDT (? failure of communication/motivation). Some ill feeling when this was apparent. KN felt he was pursuing staff for a clear answer. This then seemed also to be present in the 9.30 meeting with a lack of closure and disempowerment of the community by the community especially around time limits for selection which could drag on till 730 pm, as it had on one occasion. A compromise time agreed for meeting in second slot which ultimately seemed productive – looking at disempowerment (as above).

Informal lunch, then KN to supervision with staff and volunteers to informal meeting with residents. On account of snow etc and amid fears of train cancellation left early at 230 – rather than 330 as planned).

This visit to the new services marked the end of the first phase of the 'on the job' training. It is of interest, however, in that one of the local staff had taken the trouble to make a written record (from her perspective) of the second morning session. This was referred to in the collective diary entry above as '*Looking at breaking vicious circle of negativity by recognising positives and issue of drawing a line between junior and senior residents.*' This other subjective account can thus be compared with that of HDT. We had no knowledge that we would see this other account and ours was written before we had sight of it. The South Birmingham account, which is much richer, may shed light on what was taken from this particular session by the local team. 'Their' text appears in full below, with my subsequent comments.

Why are our residents leaving? What theories are flying around?

We had considered the possibility that the community is actively ejecting people, but when examined the individual cases of the three that left last week, we had to conclude that they made sense and that both staff and residents had worked quite hard to keep them here.

It was suggested that maybe people are leaving because it's not a very nice place to be. The original cohort may feel bereaved by all the people that have left. It was said that the recreation room is a constant reminder of the fun that was had in there in the past with people like Y and Z, when there was games and dancing. It's so hard for people to keep losing people that there is a grief hanging around.

Kingsley suggested changing the smoking rules – making the community room a smoking room and banning it in the recreation room. What would it take to make the community room a place where people wanted to be? Comfy chairs, people said. The comfy chairs were taken out of the community room and taken to the recreation room because that was a place that felt comfortable. Parallels were drawn to the two upstairs staff rooms. It was observed that all the comfy chairs have gone into the small staff room, which is a parallel process.

Main House staff asked HDT how they saw us as a staff team six months down the line from opening. HDT said that we seemed very depressed, a far cry from the enthusiasm they saw before we opened. They also said that they only get a snapshot so it's hard to be accurate. They said that we seem very stuck and it is painful to watch from the outside. There was a parallel process drawn between the issue of the senior residents that the residents are working through and our hierarchy issues. The HDT had suggested to the residents that they have a cut off point after which people become senior so as to make it not just the 'fab four' (Resident Reps plus General Secretary) who carry that. They asked whether a parallel solution might be available for the staff team.

Staff talked about the longness and nastiness of the long day shift. There was some discussion of the fact that although a lot of residents had stayed this weekend there had been very little conversation. HDT said that maybe we needed to adjust the microscope in order to see the very small but nevertheless positive changes that are happening. To stay here, and sit around a table together may be an important step for some residents. What happens in handover. So we only handover the crisis or do we handover positive stuff as well?

We talked of the importance of preserving staff sanity. Staff need to do things that they enjoy during the long day shifts even if they have to do on their own and bring stuff in. It is important that we enjoy our time here at the weekend because that is modelling something important. Not just being here because we're paid to be.

COMMENT

This account from the local patch might reveal something of the process and essence of the HDT in its relationship to the developing TCs, here mainly the staff sub-system, and in Birmingham. Many points emerge, some of which can be dissected and developed both to highlight relevant learning topics and to illustrate how the process may have been more or less successful in facilitating or inducing learning.

'*Looking at breaking vicious circle of negativity by recognising positives and issue of drawing a line between junior and senior residents*' is the HDT's summary of the above passage, which is reproduced verbatim except for the omission of the names of residents who might otherwise be identifiable.

Our words '*looking at*' imply that we were in fact trying to provide an opportunity to reflect on what had happened from a neutral position – attempting to avoid conveying views of 'right or wrong'. At various points in this local account, it was clear that what we had said was often taken as a clear suggestion, if not directive, to change, for example, with respect to the smoking rules and the recreation room. We had tried to make our offerings, however, in the spirit of possible solutions that might be considered rather than (or as much as) particular answers to particular problems.

HDT had felt they had identified a negative cycle with such aspects being dwelt upon to the exclusion of positives, hence the suggestion to consider marking positives. So we did use suggestions concretely at least some of the time! It is difficult to know now whether we had been critical in describing the staff team as 'depressed', in marked contrast to their former enthusiastic selves. It is certainly not clear how a staff member who had not been present – for whom this summary was primarily and thoughtfully prepared – might have perceived this observation made by HDT, which had been in response to a direct question.

Reading this summary now strikes the author as a mixture of South Birmingham's youth and maturity, thoughtfulness and concreteness, pessimism and optimism. Maybe all of these were present and mixed together at the time or maybe not. HDT was faced with what they perceived to be a disempowered staff team who might easily become dependent, inappropriately, on HDT rather than recognising that, as a team themselves with the residents, they might be able to solve the stated problem – 'Why are our residents leaving [early]?' HDT's making of suggestions may have felt like the dangling a tasty morsel of food in front of the mouth of a starving child but keeping it out of reach – very tantalising, perhaps at times verging on the sadistic. However, HDT very often felt powerless to help those staff who came to the sessions even though 'helping', i.e. removing their difficulties ourselves, was not exactly what we were there to do!

Maturity was there in the recognition of the sense of bereavement that arose out of so many leaving, often in unplanned and impulsive ways, with little opportunity to say goodbye. Commenting that there seemed to be parallels between what was happening 'downstairs' (in the residents' subgroup) and 'upstairs' (in the staff subgroup) was obviously too tempting for HDT to resist. 'Parallel processes' are often seen in institutions such as TCs, if one is sensitised to them. One of the clinically useful aspects of this phenomenon is the light they throw on a problematic system that is not easy to understand from a dynamic perspective. In this instance, what was obvious, once it was mentioned, was that the residents and staff were, without planning consciously to do so, acting in similar ways. Each sub-system had a newly furnished large room – spacious, light, even south-facing – and each had a smaller and dingier alternative. The 'street credible' elements of both systems took to the latter, only visiting the other on official business. In that sense, business and pleasure were being kept apart, with unhelpful consequences.

Keeping such functions separate is no sin. There are plenty of good reasons for so doing. The HDT session had brought the similarity – potential parallel processes – to light and invited those present in the session to consider whether this were merely a chance occurrence or if it meant something – an image relating to the state of the TC itself. Considering this possibility might mean that the two systems could see similarities between them and not just suffer the obvious differences and resultant difficulties. However, no such positive outcome is evident from the local report.

'*Drawing a line between junior and senior staff*' was also commented on by HDT. The usefulness of this was again identified as representing a parallel process, in this case a similar dilemma that might be capable of being dealt with by considering how the Henderson model operates. However, at Henderson (already over 50 years old) there was an obvious spread of lengths of employment within it – from 20 years to a few months. By contrast, such an informal hierarchy was lacking, at least to a large degree, at South Birmingham. Therefore, although there were staff differences in terms of role, there was very little spread in terms of longevity in familiarisation with the model. The senior staff were not necessarily more 'senior' in this important respect. People do not learn at the same rate, and there was no guarantee that those with greater overall experience and richness in previous training terms were necessarily going to learn the new method the fastest. In fact, it might be predicted that the opposite would be the case. Certainly, there was not the complexity within the new staff teams witnessed by competing hierarchies – formal and 'length of stay' – as at Henderson.

At Henderson, new staff learn much via an apprenticeship experience. They are cushioned, if not cocooned, at least to an extent, in their first year of service, by being part of a weekly new staff training group and a weekly supervision, devoted exclusively to their needs as new staff in the institution. By contrast, all the staff in the new services were, by definition, new. It was impossible therefore to reproduce the Henderson system for acculturation within the new services, at least in an authentic manner. Indeed, the HDT visits represented our attempt to do so! We represented the 'older' staff and, thinking about this dynamically, we almost certainly set in place a situation of potential rivalry between ourselves and the designated senior staff in the new services – the 'managers'.

The residents' system is deliberately set up at Henderson to represent a hierarchy based on length of stay, hence familiarity with the model of treatment, albeit a transitory and regularly changing (monthly) formal hierarchy. Again, this was impossible to do in a truly genuine manner, right at the start of this project. Opening the new residential services, everybody was 'new'. No wonder it was difficult to discern differences between a senior and junior sub-system within the resident group. Yet the establishment of this is central to the method, based as it is on Max Jones's seminal observation, that those further on in their psycho-educational programme were better teachers than the professionals alone (Jones 1952).

I recall HDT members at times feeling resentful of the dependency on them of the new staff team, feeling they were being asked to provide the support that the local seniors and managers should be providing. Looking back, we had probably not defined our own role sufficiently clearly to enable us to suffer this with more forbearance. It would seem that we were often experienced as critical, if not hyper-critical, authority figures. It is not surprising therefore that we were not always expected or welcomed, if this is what we stood for in their minds – a formal inspectorate bent on finding fault. We were often not able to stand back from this, in spite of our having set up for ourselves a supervision structure to look at our own dynamics. These sessions tended to focus defensively on staff–Volunteer relation-ships rather than on inter-staff issues, which might have led to a more meaningful understanding of ourselves in our role with the new staff teams. But often the HDT staff could not get to supervision because of the need to staff the Henderson, which was going through a series of particularly painful difficulties at the time. Was this related to the enterprise or not? Nobody could know for sure.

It might have been difficult for the new staff to hear our exhortation (or per-mission to them) to 'enjoy' their time at work. However, residents have often not endured sufficient experiences of being with those who really want them around and who want to be with them – for reasons other than a power motive, to take advantage or exploit. Therefore to provide a different experience can foster a re-evaluation of the residents' relationships. In as much as staff are experienced as being at work simply for the money, no new learning is possible. Being told to enjoy yourself may not be helpful. However, the new staff often wanted definite answers. HDT's role was to support their capacity to think rather than to rely on memory of orders given. Achieving this state of affairs, like many other aspects of the project, was easier said than done – not a case of just adding water!

Conclusions

It is accurate to say that the HDT was more preoccupied and impressed by the negative findings than by the 'positives' of replication up to the six-month point. Most of the time, we had felt ambivalently regarded by those in the new services. Perhaps this was inevitable. However, HDT's brief was one of support rather than censure, so it was perhaps not helpful in the pursuing of our task for us to have been thus preoccupied. Together, overall, we had indeed achieved so much. Although the services had opened later than expected (and too close in time to be comfortable for HDT), nobody could have known that we would ever have got that far.

By six months, both of the new residential services had the basic structural elements in place – community meetings, referred meetings, elected posts for residents, including 'Top Three'/'Resident Representatives'. So perhaps it was the culture and the articulation of the parts making up the whole that was (relatively) lacking, deficits on which HDT had tended to dwell. In particular, there did not seem to be adequate processing by Top Three and night-staff of the previous day's events, or sufficient planning of the next day's community meeting's agenda. Staff also struggled to see residents and themselves as 'groups', i.e. sub-systems within systems, interacting with other TC systems. In addition, hierarchies both between staff and residents and within the staff team appeared to be much steeper than at Henderson. HDT's training prior to the opening of the services and during visits had not enabled sufficient incorporation of these key cultural ingredients. (Indeed, it had only become clear that such were in fact key aspects with the failure of these new services to enact them. Had we had this knowledge prior to the replication project we would have placed more emphasis on these aspects in the training we delivered.)

There was clearly much anxiety in the mix – on all sides. Therefore it was not surprising that experiencing a sense of partnership was difficult. At one point, the future of the whole project was in jeopardy (again), following internal staffing difficulties in Birmingham. These necessarily reverberated across the whole replicating system. None of us could know for sure whether the sum total of what we were experiencing and witnessing meant that the two new services were essentially on track or virtually off the radar – though we favoured the former.

CHAPTER FOUR

Second Helpings

Introduction

'Replication Meetings' had been set up, under the auspices of the Steering Group, on account of the need for a separate 'structure'. These meetings reported to the Steering Group, as indeed did the HDT itself. The active life of the meetings was from May 2000 to end of March 2002. This current chapter outlines the important points that emerged during the course of these meetings and attempts to capture essential elements in the debate about what were, and what were not, agreed to be the requirements of the replication brief.

Along the way, differences of opinion emerged, especially as summarised accounts of HDT's visits to the new services were reported. Some of the records, detailing the relevant items that were departures from the Henderson model, are quoted to give the reader a flavour of the precise content of debate and to indicate the nature of formal record-keeping during this period. However, the style of the debate is not easy to infer from this source. (The time covered in this chapter overlaps with that of the last chapter and of some others.)

Early discussions

The plan was for these meetings to take place twice every three months (articulating with the quarterly Steering Group meetings) from 11.00 a.m. to 2.30 p.m. and rotating across the three sites – London, Birmingham and Crewe. The membership of the group was agreed as including the Clinical Directors and Lead Nurses from the three services together with a single representative from HDT and the Project Manager. (This meant an unbalanced membership (in favour of Henderson), which otherwise had been envisaged as being 'equal'. In total there were four members from Henderson (including the HDT and Project Manager) and two each from the other two services.) After a few meetings it was decided that there would be a regular, informal (unstructured and un-minuted) discussion to form the first part of the meeting, to facilitate discussion about 'stresses, strains, pressure-points, creative developments and collaborative working arrangements'.

Initially, the main items for the formal part of the meeting were decision-making and the 'shift system' to be adopted. However, the list grew quickly, especially after the units opened in September 2000. Agenda items then included:

- business meetings
- meeting and staff structures
- competition/collaboration
- dependency/leadership
- night-working HDT
- clinical governance
- appraisals
- staffing and roles
- TC supervision
- external training
- mutual support.

In effect, the Replication Meeting formalised the interface between HDT and the senior staff of the two new services. This was important, not least because such staff were not always present when HDT visited the sites and because already there were signs of 'splits' (senior/junior staff) developing within the staff teams. Acknowledging that HDT was, to an extent, caught up in these meant that it was important that an airing of the relevant issues could take place with senior staff alone. However, from the perspective of HDT, the views expressed by 'seniors' were often hard to reconcile with those of the 'juniors' received back at the local implementation sites. (What was still lacking was a forum at which all three groupings were represented – HDT, new TC leaders and the wider staff team/resident sub-systems.) During the second part of the January 2001 Replication Meeting – four months post-opening – it was agreed that the meetings would be chaired in turn by the local hosting staff. The main items for the agenda that month centred on:

- the remit of the Replication Meeting
- HDT feedback and
- establishing the agenda for 'Umbrella Meetings'.

The Replication Meeting's aim was to support the service replication among the three services. However it was also recognised that, in the process of achieving this, relevant clinical governance issues would necessarily be encountered. The relevant issues would be further discussed at the three-monthly Steering Groups. It was agreed that some aspects of differences among the three services would be discussed at the next Replication Meeting, in particular, staffing and management structures.

Setting up of the first Umbrella Meeting was also agreed. Birmingham would host the inaugural meeting on 7 February and Henderson would set the agenda, following discussion with the other services. A total of 56 people would be accommodated, approximately 15 to 20 from each service. The meeting would start at half past ten (with coffee) and end (with tea) at four o'clock. This would turn out to be a tiring day, given the long distance that needed to be travelled by most parties. The residential 'lead' consultant from Henderson (Alex Esterhuyzen) was leading the organisation of the Umbrella Meeting's agenda rather than myself. This was to include and involve non-HDT staff, so that some of the rifts between this subgroup of Henderson staff and HDT might be healed. It was envisaged that the occasion would enable 'catch-up' for all staff with respect to the service development. The overall aim of the Umbrella Meetings was for the three service elements to meet to start to become one service, as well as to provide some informal time for social exchange and mutual 'peer' education, à la Maxwell Jones.

HDT feedback included a discussion of the next phase (six to twelve months post-opening) of the visits to the new services and it was agreed that the dates for all of these would be circulated. The future role of the Volunteers was also discussed and how their involvement would need to be phased out. At this point it should be noted there was still a plan to involve current Henderson residents, although this decision was subsequently revoked. It is perhaps of interest to note that in the Replication Meeting in Birmingham on 14 March 2001 there were prominent issues to do with internal TC finances, mostly not related to replication:

- residents' access to budgets

- hotel accommodation to be funded by local service and travel costs via the host service

- information about the payments to service users

- working with ex-service users and residents' employment

- selection process audit.

However, the main item for this meeting concerned the management structures within the three services and how these related to their respective Trust's over-arching management structures. It was acknowledged that some of these structures had changed considerably since the start of the replication project, without this being explicitly discussed; hence their implications had not been properly taken into account. Each service therefore outlined its current internal management structure and discussed its relationship to its own Trust Board. One of the action points resulting from this was the decision to circulate (to the Consultant Lead and Nurse Lead of the other two services) the minutes of each service's main business meeting. (This was an attempt to integrate the service into a single entity, as well as to support replication.) It is of interest to note that in Crewe the Webb House management structure seemed to be closest to that of the Henderson when the replication project had started. The irony, however, was that Webb House was now different from the other two services in respect of the proximity of its link to senior levels within its hosting Trust.

A financial issue, which became a long-running item, was that to do with Social Therapists' pay. It had emerged (possibly through the informal discussions occurring at the first Umbrella Meeting) that Social Therapists were paid different amounts across the three services. This led to understandable discontent in those staff members paid less. Although the relevant managers had a rationale for their differing positions, it was agreed that each service should exchange their pay scales, job descriptions and reasoning for the Social Therapist roles in order to facilitate a discussion at the next Replication Meeting. What was also encouraged at this March meeting (i.e. six months subsequent to the new services opening) was the desirability of staff visiting each other's services. It was envisaged that this would allow closer links to be made. In particular, it was thought to be useful for Webb House and Main House staff to visit one another, so as to further the cause of replication, through identifying both similarities and differences. (The geographical distance between Crewe and Birmingham is relatively small.)

This March 2001 Replication Meeting coincided with the start of 'Phase 2' of the HDT visits. The original plan, for this phase, had been to have fortnightly visits during the ensuing period of six months. It represented a halving of the frequency of the visits. Travelling difficulties, however, had made it necessary to change the original format of visits into two-day blocks, occurring at half the originally envisaged frequency. (Although no comment is made to this effect, my memory has it that these two-day blocks, in being less onerous in terms of travel, had been welcomed by HDT, perhaps an indirect marker of fatigue setting in.) Even though the size of input was essentially similar to that originally agreed for HDT's visits, the distance between 'samplings' was increased (i.e. to monthly rather than fortnightly). It is impossible to know what effect this 'dilution' might have had. There were pros as well as cons to having an extended (i.e. two-day) period of visiting the new services. On the plus side, there was the potential for HDT to be better absorbed within the TC and consequently less distorting of that which it was observing. On the minus side, HDT was worse placed to pick up variations in atmosphere of the new TCs through visiting half as often – only two days per month per site, during this second six months post-opening.

Dangerous disagreement

What is also of considerable interest, in perusing the minutes of this March 2001 Replication Meeting, is the opaque comment that '*HDT provided some feedback about Webb House and Main House*'. My memory is that we did not wish the detailed content discussed to be conveyed more widely. The reasons for this are complex. There was often a mutual avoidance of confrontation within these meetings, and HDT certainly were reticent about feeding back very negative aspects to our opposite numbers. I recall feeling caught in a situation of divided loyalties – to the wider staff team of the local services on the one hand and to their senior colleagues – my immediate peers – on the other. In neither forum were both parties present and uncomfortable 'splitting' was rife, as mentioned above. Certainly we were struggling to be open with one another in these Replication Meetings, even though problems that needed open and full discussion formed the reason for the creation of these meetings in the first place. A lot of the time (relative) conflict avoidance and opaque reporting seemed the best that we could manage.

It may be not unconnected to this last point that there were no Birmingham staff present at the following Replication Meeting, which took place in Sutton on 11 April 2001. One of the issues discussed was 'how unstructured time is used' within the democratic TC programme. This had been a difficulty previously highlighted by HDT, particularly in relation to Birmingham. It was felt that the importance and purpose of unstructured time was not well understood. It was agreed at this meeting to circulate a relevant academic paper and for this topic to be included at the next Umbrella Meeting. It can be seen therefore how the potential role of the 'Umbrellas' could be incorporated so as to close a kind of 'audit loop', relevant gaps having been identified by HDT or emanating from discussion at the Replication Meetings.

Also in the April 2001 Replication Meeting were discussed issues of 'bullying and power' and how these aspects might be managed within the TC. What is noted in the minutes of this meeting is the relationship between these aspects and the notion of 'permissiveness'. Ostensibly, permissiveness relates to a tolerance of attitudes and behaviour within the residents subgroup of the TC, although, arguably, it also extends to a similar phenomenon within the staff team and in relation to colleagues. Within a few months of the start of these new residential services, each had had to deal with formal complaints, of one sort or another, hence the relevance of a discussion within the Replication Meeting to see if they dealt with these by similar processes and methods, hence serving replication. Interestingly, Henderson too was in the throes of dealing with a grievance – a matter that would continue to run for many months, not least because the merger of its Trust had taken place during that time, further complicating the management of the grievance process and prolonging it. (Originally, we had not considered it necessary to replicate such processes, hence Henderson had not provided relevant policy information. Almost certainly, this had been a mistake.)

For many years at Henderson, there had been a tradition for team problems to be aired in staff meetings, resulting in 'free and frank' exchanges between staff members. These were within a formal group setting (i.e. a staff meeting) but not always with full participation of the whole group. At times, therefore, some staff would be centre stage (whether willingly or reluctantly) and others peripheral, so to speak, in the audience and as spectators. This scenario, not uncommon but not obviously healthy, had become part of Henderson's culture. The line between an in-depth discussion of inter-staff difficulties (or indeed positive aspects) and this forum serving some form of 'therapy' was sometimes blurred within these so-called 'sensitivity' meetings. Therapy was never the intended remit of this meeting, but sometimes, in effect, a staff member would be offered up as the 'sick' one, as the result of scapegoating – in spite of this meeting being facilitated by an external professional. During the course of the replication project this aspect of Henderson's practice came under Trust scrutiny and, as a result, was changed. It is now termed the 'Team Awareness Meeting' and has a clearer remit and tighter boundaries, making it a safer space and the above developments less likely to arise or persist.

Emerging consensus

Not a million miles from this issue and one also discussed in the same Replication Meeting, is that of the TC's response to a resident's law-breaking and the need for uniformity in responding to such aspects, as part of replication and as part of a single national severe PD service. The minutes refer to the fact that '*Clinicians needed to use judgement about what needed to be reported to the Police and that advice can be sought from the relevant Trust and professional bodies if necessary*'. This advice is apparently clear and straightforward. However, what was only covertly communicated was a sense of anxiety about the limits of power and responsibility of the developing TCs and the extent to which their means of dealing with such aspects might be at odds with those of more mainstream psychiatric services. In fact, all psychiatric services struggle to do justice to such aspects; for example, as to when to attempt to press charges against a patient and when not. (Meanwhile the Social Therapists' pay issue continued to rumble on, representing another aspect of the three services with which we were still struggling in order to grow into an integrated whole.)

On a more positive note, also from this same April 2001 Replication Meeting, the issues surrounding the Care Programme Approach (CPA) were discussed. South West London and St George's NHS Trust, our new Trust, was in a position to circulate its documentation in respect of CPA, which served as an example of the way in which there could be an economy of larger scale with three services operating as one. Henderson was able to help out the other services through enabling them to avoid re-inventing (the whole of) this particular wheel through a perusal of our own documentation. As a further example of mutual benefit, the circulated job descriptions of the Birmingham Social Therapist posts served as a useful template for Henderson, showing us what a 'modern' job description and person specification looked like!

In the June 2001 Replication Meeting, in Birmingham, we acknowledged the departure of our Lead Nurse (Neil Hamer) and also one of the stalwarts of the

HDT (Kevin Polley). The loss of these two staff members exemplified some of the negative events occurring within Henderson Hospital – negative in the sense of others needing to cover the gaps left by these valued colleagues (it was positive for them that they had good jobs into which to move). The number of staff vacancies at Henderson reveals something of the level of strain that Henderson was under at this point. Approximately one sixth of the total complement of posts was unfilled:

- Specialist Clinical Nurse
- Clinical Nurse Manager
- Two Social Therapists
- E Grade Nurse
- Business Manager.

Progressing a complex replication process, with a succession of individuals in the key posts, posed a problem that we encountered repeatedly. The high turnover of staff during the project may well have been related to the added stresses generated by it, though it is impossible to be sure. A spate of HDT pregnancies is harder to account for on this basis! This too contributed to the high turnover.

Given the remit of the Replication Meeting, it is not clear at this distance (nor was it at the time) why the Social Therapists' pay item continued to take centre stage. The issue was concrete and therefore potentially more solvable than some of the more ephemeral and subtle replication matters. In retrospect, the matter may have served to distract us from issues that might have been more divisive. The differences in the amounts the Social Therapists were paid in the three services caused relatively little actual division within the meeting.

Part of the HDT feedback from the June 2001 meeting was the announcement that 'workgroups' would be visited during the final phase of their visits (September 2001 to March 2002). This would necessitate a change of days (from Tuesdays/Wednesdays to Thursdays/Fridays) when HDT visited. Other feedback at this point seemed relatively optimistic, expressing the view that we were 'seeing replication'. It was also noted that in both new services the resident groups were showing signs of 'differentiation' into the newer residents and those older, who were starting to plan for their leaving. Such differentiation obviously brought the new services more into line with that of Henderson. This also served to make more relevant some of the structure and function of the TC that HDT had taken for granted would have made sense to the new services. It was only in retrospect that HDT had become aware of how difficult it was for the new services to get under way with everybody having been equally new – a situation which did not marry up with Maxwell Jones's (1952) original observation about the 'older' teaching the 'newer'. Therefore, the period of initial service development lacked something quintessential to the democratic TC, namely, the capacity of those further on to help and support those just beginning. HDT staff and ex-residents had been relatively poor substitutes.

Surprising setbacks

In the ensuing Replication Meetings, other issues were beginning to surface, some of which were surprising, if not shocking to Henderson ears. The Steering Group had agreed to develop shared documentation across the three democratic TCs in respect of inclusion and exclusion criteria. Therefore, we were surprised to hear that these had not been adhered to. Also at this meeting, Webb House declared that it was changing its programme, and in particular, decreasing the number of times per week that the small groups would meet – from three to two. This felt like a significant shift and departure from Henderson's practice, although at the meeting there was little time left to discuss the matter or raise an objection.

The Henderson staff present experienced this as a *fait accompli* and out of keeping with the spirit of collaboration that was the trademark of our project – at least our agreed aim. (Somewhat guiltily, however, I reflected that we ourselves had made a change to our in-house 'surgery' practice without having communicated this. To my mind, at least, this was of less significance than Webb's change to small groups, but nonetheless this was a departure that could and should have been communicated to them by us, if not also discussed beforehand.) An action point deriving from this was that all three services would present their current programmes for scrutiny to see how far they were actually similar and how far different!

Items that were to be discussed at future meetings included clinical governance, disability and sexual abuse. From these, looking back now, it is clear that to some extent the replication process had the effect of 'modernising' Henderson Hospital. Paradoxically, the process of replication, as well as aiming to stamp its imprint on those new services, changed Henderson Hospital. (I had privately felt before going into the replication project that Henderson was too inward-looking, but I had felt unable to change this significantly. I had hoped that, through setting up new services and then relating to a set of new colleagues, Henderson might be able to expand its somewhat narrow horizons.) In this regard, NSCAG's notion that replication was what the three of us decided it was did actually make sense.

If the June 2001 minutes conveyed a positive message with respect to replication, then a letter from me dated 4 July 2001 (see below for extract) contradicts this, at least in respect of the Birmingham service. It relates to an HDT visit there, although it found its way into my Replication Meeting folder. (Arguably, this document could have appeared in the previous chapter.)

I was concerned that neither [senior staff] were present at the Friday community meeting and feel I need to question whether there is sufficient senior support for the team, in terms of an accurate-enough replication of the Henderson model. I know that [same senior staff] are not present on Wednesdays because of the management meeting, unless this had recently been re-scheduled... To my mind, it is a trademark of the Henderson model to have at least one of the two clinical leads present at each community meeting.

My fear is that with the continuing relative absence of senior input on a daily basis, there is an impaired containment function which will hamper your efforts to increase the size of the resident group so that you have a viable 'community'. To put these comments in context, I think there will only have been a handful of occasions over the 12 years or so that I have been at Henderson, when the most senior [nursing] manager and both the consultants would have been absent from a community meeting at the same time...

I have felt impelled to put things down in writing rather than merely telephoning my concerns... I hope we can re-visit some of the above when we next meet at 'replication'...

Also in the same folder was a letter dated 13 July from the Director of Webb House. It pointed to a difficulty arising in both the new services, in relation to the appointment of the third (medical) Consultant. The original plan/suggestion/directive from Henderson was to appoint all such senior staff near to the start. Neither service in fact had done this. As a result, more than nine months after the service had been operational, not all the relevant senior staff in the new services were in post. Those who were certainly felt the resulting strain. (Initially, both new services had lacked adequate Business Manager support, and this state of affairs continued for a long period in Birmingham, presumably contributing to difficulties with recruitment.) Various effects stemmed from this lack of senior staff, including the need for existing seniors to be more thinly spread. Unfortunately, this resulted in their being away from the clinical front line and therefore unable to replicate the prominence of senior staff which obtained at Henderson, notably in the community and referred meetings (see above letter).

The effect of this senior staff situation was that 'rota staff' necessarily needed to act up for their '9 to 5' colleagues although, because of the demands and dictates of the rota, they could not provide the continuity of staffing required. To an extent other '9 to 5' staff occupied a kind of 'middle-management' tier, not seen at Henderson, to offset this. In practice, these staff were often uncomfortably caught in the middle between the actual seniors and the rota staff. All in all, this state of affairs reflected the fact that Henderson Hospital did not have the authority to impose structures, and yet it retained an equal share of total responsibility for matters when they failed to progress.

For HDT, the issue was one of dealing with feelings of impotence but also not really knowing how best to intervene in the face of problems, since in certain respects the new services had departed significantly from the Henderson model (for example, the different shift pattern in Birmingham or the twice-weekly small groups in Crewe). The greater the departure, the less was HDT's confidence and competence to diagnose and treat any subsequent/consequent 'disorder'. At the

July 2001 Replication Meeting in Crewe, major disparities in terms of the inclusion and exclusion criteria of referral to our national service were identified. All of these issues required clarification:

- disability access for wheelchairs
- people who have limited ability to self-care
- problems with visual acuity
- difficulties with hearing
- aged over 45 years
- aged 17–18 years
- people on the sexual abuser register for abuse of a minor
- referrals by GPs
- self-referrals.

As well as concerns about operating a discriminatory programme, there was also a concern about litigation resulting from our operating services that differed from that advertised – a trade descriptions issue? However, there was an acceptance that, during the initial developmental phase, there might necessarily be differences between Henderson and the two new services in terms of patients who could be accepted as appropriate referrals. As a mark of the seriousness with which these departures were taken, however, a number of action points resulted. One was that we decided that all three services should look back at our shared 'Referrer's Guide' document, which had been circulated to potential referrers. We should indicate precisely how our services departed from the stated criteria, if at all. It was also noted that an 'equity of access group' would need to be established and report back to the Steering Group. In addition, it was agreed that we should define a set of common criteria at the 'September' Replication Meeting (for reasons of annual leave, to be held on 3 October 2001).

Safer territory

In October, at this next meeting, it was proposed that we look at the organisation of the three services, from the perspective of the Replication Meeting, to consider obstacles to the three services integrating as a single national service, given their differing Trust structures. It was also noted that there was a need to consider how the services might be influenced by the differential functioning of their Outreach component. As a result of the ensuing discussion, a whole day's meeting was proposed, with an external facilitator who could bring a 'systems orientation' to the process. This was a crucial step. With hindsight, however, although appropriately forward-looking (anticipating the end of the 18 months' development phase at the end of March 2002), I have a suspicion that we had been glossing over important differences in our hastening towards unification. Certainly we were to enter some choppy water with respect to this study day.

The timing of this 3 October Replication Meeting also marked both the passage of the first anniversary of the new services being operational and entry to the last six months of the 'set-up' period. HDT feedback in the meeting commented that the Volunteers had completed their input as a core part of the team and that this had been marked by 'affectionate goodbyes from Main House and Webb House'. It was also reported that there were some plans for current residents at Henderson to arrange to meet their peers in Birmingham and Crewe – though this was to take many months to actualise. There was even a discussion of some kind of 'Umbrella equivalent' for residents, across the three services, although it was noted that money would need to be identified to support such a venture. Parsimoniously, it was suggested that just the 'Top Three' residents from each service might meet together – a cheaper option.

It was also clarified at this meeting that HDT would carry on in their existing format of two-day meetings and therefore only be visiting each site three times, in the final six months. The pros and cons of such a plan were acknowledged (as above). It was noted that there would be no HDT contact with residents, not least since none of the new residents would have been known to HDT, given the lack of the latter's involvement in pre-selection and preparatory activities. Also the nature of the visits would necessarily change and might include role-playing and the reading of scientific papers. The plan was for particular topics to be discussed and for local staff to select these topics. This was to acknowledge the increasing equality between the two new services and Henderson.

It was noted that there had been a 'round-up meeting' between HDT staff and Volunteers on 25 September 2001. The minutes of this meeting were to be circulated to Birmingham and Crewe. In particular they emphasised important issues, which had been hard to rectify, to do with:

- entering and leaving the community

- encouraging group interaction, especially in community meetings

- processing the previous day's business in community meetings

- establishing a formal resident hierarchy.

The implication of this minute is that the aspects applied equally to both new services. This was not actually the case. However, there were similarities, which suggests that such aspects, in being problematic to embed, were not only intrinsically difficult but also crucial to the therapeutic ingredients within the TC mix, i.e. those that needed to be replicated.

It was reported that the forthcoming study day was discussed again and the invitation list agreed namely as: three Outreach members; three Lead Nurses; three Directors and three Business Managers. The easy symmetry of this list defies the difficulties that continued to exercise all of us, which was to harmonise inclusion and exclusion criteria of admissions to the three services. The idea of the three working as one, which we had all readily signed up to at the start of this project, was much more difficult to deliver in practice. An agreement was forged that:

> The three units would need to work as one service to negotiate and take points/arguments for extending the upper age limit and possibly lowering the lower age limit back to NSCAG. This would be via the Steering Group which includes the Directors of each service and representation from the Chief Executives.

The advisory nature of the Replication Meetings is clear from this note, which distinguished it from the Steering Group that had (limited) power to take executive action.

The effect of shifting the September meeting to 3 October meant that the next Replication Meeting followed only one week later. (For two successive meetings the regular Birmingham membership was absent, hence deputies had been supplied.) One of the main items discussed, again, was the planned study day and we agreed to discuss the following issues:

- What we are aiming to become, how we are going to get there and the time-scale this will take.

- To be clear about the interface with the Steering Group.

- HDT is going, what will take its place?

- Interface with the Association of Therapeutic Communities and perhaps other groups.

- What will tie us together?

What is clear from the action point resulting from this meeting was the extent to which the tasks were already being shared among the three services, so that even though the planned meeting to discuss a unified service had not happened, there was a sense of a growing and effective collaboration among the three partners. Given the importance of the 'unification', I enclose a copy of the draft programme for the study day (Figure 4.1), which the external facilitator negotiated with the three Directors. However, in our looking forward to the final phase of the setting-up process, it was as if all the messiness of the development phase could be simply swept under the carpet and that we could sail confidently into a shared and integrated future. But we did not.

Also in the service of promoting unification, there is a letter on file from the South Birmingham Director (27 November 2001), which outlines one possible way forward for the sharing of important tasks. This is another example of the way in which the siren of unification beckoned us as if into safer water. The

---

EXTENDED REPLICATION MEETING: DRAFT TASK AND PROGRAMME
Tuesday and Wednesday, 11, 12th December 2001

	Tuesday, 11th December
1.00	Lunch together
2.00	**Setting-up: Moving on** An opening session to acknowledge the road travelled by the services over the past year or so. It will enable a celebration of progress and taking stock of the need to 'move on' after a setting-up period. Discussion of key future objectives for individual centres and collectively.
3.30	Tea
3.45	**Loose-tight (1): Clinical Practice** An assessment of what are key common (tight) characteristics of clinical practice (residential and Outreach) for the future of the service. A time limited discussion to draw out the key characteristics and identification of further work. This could shape the organisational arrangements – hence its position in the programme.
Short break	
5.15	**Loose-tight (2): Issues for organisational arrangements** What key 'tight' characteristics are necessary for the service to be adequately organised in its administration and finance, e.g. meeting structures, delegated authority. Issues and proposals.
6.30	Finish
7.30	Dinner

	Wednesday, 12th December
9.00	**Loose-tight (3): Agreeing organisational arrangements** Discussion and committing to organisational arrangements. This may include new delegations and forms.
10.30	Coffee/Tea
10.45	**Loose-tight (4): External relationships** The service has hugely complex 'external' relationships. What tight characteristics are necessary for clinical practice, administration and finance across the three centres in relation to their external environment.
12.00	**Taking stock/Action Plans** Agreement as to what, who and by when action needs to take place.
1.00	Lunch together and depart.

Figure 4.1 Draft programme for the study day

suggestion was that one service should lead on each of the following: continuing professional development, clinical governance, finance, equity of access, and research. Meanwhile, the Crewe Director was taking the lead on the agenda for this meeting, which proved to be enjoyable and productive and is set out in the Appendix as summarised by the external facilitator.

The Replication Meeting then seems to go into a bureaucratic overdrive with the identification of tasks to be completed by 9 January 2002:

- propose a name for the successor of the Steering Group
- decide how the Chair is appointed
- agree a proposal for membership of the community
- address issues about future agendas
- consider the impact of this new group on existing management groups
- define the terms of reference and review the notes made on 11–12 December (facilitated study day).

At the Replication Meeting of 9 January 2002 it was agreed that there was a need to be '*pro-active in formulating a proposal for a new structure for the National Service that will initially be agreed with NSCAG and subsequently negotiated with the three Trusts*'. In fact, this was to turn out to be a stumbling block, and our new national structure was never formally ratified or even recognised within any of the three respective Trusts. Nevertheless, we were still buoyed up sufficiently to name the new group – 'National Service Management Group' (NSMG). We appointed the Chair (Keith Hyde, nominated by Jan Birtle, seconded by me and agreed unanimously by all present). We also agreed to advise NSCAG formally that we would be dissolving the Steering Group following the February 2002 meeting and that the NSMG would be inaugurated at that time. Beyond this point the content of my Replication Meetings folder does not extend.

Conclusions

It may seem odd, since the essence of this project was to 'replicate' Henderson, that a specific regular meeting needed to be instigated to define replication and to maintain our steady progress towards this goal. Suffice it to say, it proved necessary for those of us associated with the project at a senior level to meet separately to attempt to agree what we believed replication to be. As indicated in Chapter 1, we had not been successful in finding TC literature from which to extract a precise recipe that we could follow. At Henderson we knew about running an 'elderly' service, though not a brand new or developing one. We ourselves, therefore, did not have all the necessary expertise. Neither could we know what a service destined to become a replica would look like at a given developmental stage. Nor could those actually running the new services know that they were on the correct replication trajectory. It was thus a matter of trust and faith in one another to discuss and disagree, if necessary, but also to find agreement as to what amounted to replication, at a particular stage.

We did not know for sure which structural ingredients of Henderson (if any) could be dispensed with, without adversely affecting the essential culture. The relevant experiments simply had not been and could not be done. However, the values and practices of the modern NHS could not allow a simple and total replication, even if desired by all the replication participants. With respect to this, HDT felt that some of the senior staff in the new services were relieved that they could not be expected to replicate Henderson completely – perhaps an uncharitable or inaccurate view. However, in many of these Replication Meetings, we found it hard to be open with one another. In denying differences of opinion, therefore, we were creating, in effect, an inauthentic alliance and thwarting a genuine partnership. To an extent, issues such as the Social Therapists' pay were spurious and served to distract us from areas of real difference that needed confronting – namely, those tentatively identified by HDT. We never really found out, however, why HDT's suggestions were so difficult to take up. It was as if this were too dangerous a topic for us to confront.

The temptation to get beyond the developmental stage – to become a system of three equal TCs and a single national service – seemed irresistible. We all wanted it but, perhaps unconsciously, believed that it could only be achieved if we feigned our unity via indulging in a bureaucratic exercise that ultimately delivered only the shell of a structure – the National Service Management Group – that had no authority vested in it locally, let alone nationally. Having said this, the strength of our partnership in delivering two new functioning services should not be denied.

CHAPTER FIVE

Aftertaste

Introduction

The replication bid, originally produced by five Trusts, including South Birmingham and Mental Health Services of Salford (MHSS), had represented a shared blueprint of how together we might proceed, assuming the bid to NSCAG were successful. However, the idea of a partnership and its reality are seldom the same, as we were all repeatedly to discover. The purpose of this chapter therefore is to provide a retrospective view of tensions and dissent – subtle or overt, indirect or direct – that sometimes soured our relationships as we encountered difficulties with replicating.

This chapter considers some potential early influences – witting or unwitting, individual or collective – that contributed to the reality of the collaborative endeavour. The detailed content, including all the factual material, derives from contemporaneous records and correspondence. As most of this emanated from the Steering Group of which I was Chair, it might be challenged over what is 'fact' and what 'opinion', although the minutes of the relevant meetings were duly scrutinised for accuracy, in the time-honoured fashion. With this issue in mind, however, I try to convey where the written account was at odds with the views of some others and where it had been difficult to reach agreement.

The Steering Group, initially, was to be a bi-monthly event. The first one took place in Birmingham (6 November 1997), the plan being for the venue of this meeting to rotate around the three different sites, relating to the national service. It should be noted, however, that at the outset there were no identified premises for the new services. Meeting venues were thus in a variety of existing mental health service provisions. Note also that, at this time, no funding was in fact available from NSCAG. This did not start until April 1998. Thus all the work undertaken until that time derived from the existing resources of the participating NHS Trusts, not an inconsiderable amount – though never actually calculated or costed. Although there had been a loss of momentum occasioned by the protracted decision-making involved (six months), the Steering Group came together promptly and began to compose itself.

At its first meeting (of 14 people, with no apologies) we introduced ourselves. As Chair, I rehearsed briefly – well, fairly briefly – the history of the bid and relevant Henderson 'pre-history' leading up to the decision to tender. The first item of business records that 'The NSCAG committee had asked for the bid to reflect the financial restraints for 1998/9 [and] this resulted in a changed action plan'. We were starting how we would go on, though at this stage we could not know this – the goalposts were on the move! Much would not go according to plan and this would bring repeated disappointment and a searching for people – internal and external to our partnership – to blame for this!

Relative strangers and early conversations

At the start, the Steering Group comprised relative strangers. Although collaborating on this project, we rarely met other than to do this business. Aside from working for the NHS, we had only the replication project in common and few casual meetings or informal contacts that might have helped to build better relationships and in turn form a more secure platform on which to develop mutual respect and trust. So, an early test of mutuality was NSCAG's requirement for us to start more gradually than planned, 'to reflect the financial constraints'. Although initially frustrated by this, their requirement gave us more time to sort ourselves out. The large size and considerable complexity of the collaborative task, therefore, had more time to dawn on us – pennies were dropping, in more ways than one. Though less than anticipated, the total funding available for 1998/99 was approximately £2.5 million. This represented the costs of the existing Henderson service and start-up monies for the two new services, all of which was channelled via Henderson (then still part of St Helier NHS Trust). The bid would not be funded fully until April 1999.

In this first Steering Group meeting, the duration of NSCAG funding was referred to as being three years. There was no documentation of any dissent or discussion of this matter (and the minutes were religiously copied to NSCAG). As I recall, few of us saw the project as actually capable of delivery, including on the mandatory independent research of the process, within such a short period. The submitted plan required the full staff complement to have been recruited and inducted for 'Site 1' to open in March 1999 and 'Site 2' three months later. The new services were referred to in this way since nobody knew which would obtain their premises first and hence attract the lion's share of the set-up money in Year 1 of the funding. (These milestones could no longer stand given the delay in full funding and would be re-calculated, not for the last time.) Also in this inaugural meeting, the Steering Group concluded, 'The identification of appropriate premises was likely to be the key driver for deciding how the different sites would be phased.' None of us could have imagined, in the excitement of this first meeting, how slow would be the progress on securing suitable premises. Without knowing it, we were in for a very long and slow 'drive'.

Under an item simply entitled 'Funding', it was noted that 'the funding was expected to be longer term [i.e. longer than three years] as the NSCAG committee was suggesting a possible addition to the number of sites as originally identified in the application'. At this point, we were unsure whether unspent monies could be held over from one financial year to the next. Given the developmental nature of this service replication project we were hopeful that they could. However, the answer we obtained subsequently was a firm 'no'. This would lead to a series of troublesome negotiations.

It was noted that South Birmingham Mental Health NHS Trust 'was currently making strategic decisions about the future of psychotherapy services and these would be influenced by the requirements of the new services'. This was an indirect way of saying that redundancies (which the Trust presumably for financial as well as other reasons preferred not to create) were planned but could be avoided were alternative employment – this project – to be identified. This factor is relevant in terms of the influence of the local history. This was referred to in the organisational researcher's report (see Chapter 6), though she was not to be in post until January 1999, i.e. later than this note of 1997. Essentially, this project provided South Birmingham with an additional, if not primary, motive for pursuing the replication project.

Before the second Steering Group meeting (7 January 1998), bearing in mind the 'local history' point just made, I received a letter from a senior medical member of the South Birmingham Trust indicating delight at our good fortune in securing the successful NSCAG bid and stressing the need for 'dedicated staff' in order to 'match the time-scale' of the project. These were both eminently reasonable points to make, but the letter went on to indicate that a local Consultant had been identified and that the Chief Executive 'wishes to invite X to fulfil this post'. It was trusted what such arrangements might meet with my approval and my views were looked forward to, 'in due course'. This apparently polite suggestion represented what was to become a stumbling block, serving to divide the Steering Group, for a number of months, especially its medical members and especially the South Birmingham Trust, from Henderson/St Helier NHS Trust.

The process of being divided was painful to all concerned, coming as it did so early on in the process of collaboration. We were all anxious and suspicious of one another, as well as excited – the heady mix of new relationships. At times it led to ill-feeling that might have jeopardised the success of the overall project. It is possible that emotional scars still persist today. How far such injury also served to promote subsequent disagreements is not possible to know. My objections to a purely local appointment seemed to serve to convey mistrust in the available local skills and talents, which was not, and is not, the case. But there were to be more adversarial exchanges, and not simply between South Birmingham and Henderson Hospital.

The second Steering Group meeting also took place in Birmingham; perhaps this was the least difficult place for all to reach. However, the faded, but still grand, surroundings of the Uffculme Clinic (once home to the Cadbury family) probably also exerted its attraction. At this meeting it was confirmed, via NSCAG's communication, that the initial bid documentation did represent 'a full business case'. There had been a worry that we might have been required to provide still more detailed plans, which we felt would merely have delayed matters further. The momentum seemed to be building again.

The original timetable of project milestones had been circulated, and the minutes stated that 'any changes to these timetables should be realistic and should be agreed by all concerned'. Reading this now, the note seems to convey authority and clarity. However, as a Steering Group, we would not be able to assert such authority, even when we were unanimous in our views. Mention is made of contributing to the development of forensic psychotherapy (July 1998), part of the original thinking and reflecting the important work done on 'difficult and offender patients' represented in the Reed Report, on the back of which came our successful bid to NSCAG. (This aspect, which is peripheral to the replication project, was in fact partially successful. Two specialist registrar posts in forensic psychotherapy were set up – in South Birmingham and South West London and St George's Mental Health NHS Trust – out of seven that had been agreed nationally. A large amount of time was consumed by this endeavour.)

Premises, premises

A new timetable was generated and funding estimates made, as well as estimates of our projected Year 1 activity. It was reiterated that the premises were to be afforded priority over everything else. We also decided that no staff could be appointed until we had premises. Yet this decision put us in a 'Catch 22' situation, since without more staff dedicated to the project, i.e. having it as their main job, we would be less likely to find suitable accommodation and to find it soon. The clock of NSCAG's (potentially) time-limited funding had started ticking in April 1998. After that, at some point, the research-funding clock would also add its 'tock'. Both added to the strain that the Steering Group were under.

Whichever service found its accommodation first would have the larger share of the first year's set-up money, but the 'second' service would need to follow on closely behind, lest the gap got too large for the constraints imposed by the respective (time-limited) ticking cash-clocks to accommodate. For both the service development and research plans to work out, both new services needed to be closely in phase with one another! A wider separation would also make a more prolonged drain on the Henderson Hospital resource devoted to the project. All in all, we needed to develop quickly, but then, as we were to experience repeatedly, we were not in a position to dictate the pace of development. The 'premises' were firmly established in the driving seat!

In our Steering Group minutes, it was noted that NSCAG had 'indicated that funding was likely to be for a period longer than the initial three year period, although it was thought to be unlikely that this could be confirmed in writing from NSCAG, since the development is subject to annual review in line with NSCAG policy'. We had hoped to have something in writing, since its absence added risk (and stress) to the enterprise of Trusts allocating resources (financial and human) to a project that might be of so short a duration. Managing this financial risk factor a few months later on was indirectly to account for a delay of several months.

It was already anticipated by the time of the second Steering Group meeting that the effect of European Union legislation could add undesirable delays to the planned time-scale, since developing a partnership, for example with a housing association, to commission suitable premises involved a cumbersome bureaucratic process. Even at this early stage of the project, Birmingham reported that it had already 'corresponded with over 100 potential contacts for a building in the West Midlands'. Sadly, little was to come of such intense activity for well over a year. Ironically, Henderson's decision to prioritise partnerships with Birmingham and Greater Manchester had rested, among other things, on the large populations represented and, erroneously as it turned out, the large number of suitable premises potentially available.

We reminded ourselves in the handsome Uffculme Clinic (coveted but unaffordable, on account of its being unsafe accommodation for patients) that 'the remit of the Outreach Service should cover pre – and post-treatment and provide a supervisory and training function'. For Henderson, this represented a change that, among a number of others, was not entirely welcomed (and would lead to internal divisions). On the one hand, Henderson's Outreach function was expanding in terms of numbers of staff. On the other hand, its catchment area, originally simply the South-West Thames Region, had more than quadrupled. Added to this its therapeutic remit was diluted, to become only a 'before and after' Henderson service. The addition of staff to service the new Outreach function also meant that new and larger accommodation had to be found.

Details of the recruitment of the 'core team' of the new services were discussed in this January 1998 meeting. The discussion was inconclusive but formed a crucial debate whose implications were potentially far-reaching. The plan was to revisit this issue at the March 1998 meeting. The format of this next meeting, which was to be held in Sutton, was to be extended to incorporate a discussion with Henderson staff and also with staff and residents together – the first formal involvement of service users. The aim was for Henderson to present what they saw as the key TC principles that would form the basis for replication. A number of ideological and pragmatic aspects were to be covered:

- liaison with local services
- relationship with the Trust
- care programme approach
- community relations
- management function of clinicians
- description of the resident group

- decision-making

- ethnicity issues.

With the residents also present, two particular issues were discussed – resident involvement and decision-making in the democratic TC. Lunch followed in the Sutton Hospital Restaurant – a forgettable event. The formal Steering Group continued after lunch, from 1.45 to 4 p.m.

The detail of the available money for setting up in Year 1 had been communicated – £577,800 and £216,300. In this meeting, South Birmingham stated they would need additional capital to refurbish any building – though we all knew there was no separate identified money – and it was suggested that approaches be made elsewhere (i.e. not the NHS) to obtain this. MHSS (Salford) reported they had placed an advertisement in the *Official Journal of the European Union* for partners to fund premises and had received eight responses. They also indicated they wished to involve Henderson residents in progressing this venture. At this point, MHSS seemed to us to be working within the TC ethos, involving a spirit of deep collaboration – 'communalism' – more so than South Birmingham.

St Helier NHS Trust's advice to South Birmingham on its Director appointment, a matter now starting to grumble on, had been that it should be made through a national advertisement. The process was outlined in the NHS Consultant Appointments Guidelines, which we were finally able to track down. This stated that:

> Where, exceptionally, an employing body wishes to make an appointment without advertising the post, the application to the Secretary of State should include a detailed statement of the circumstances giving rise to the application, a CV of the applicant concerned and details of local professional support of the application…in all cases…employing bodies must still ensure that an AAC is convened to consider the applicant's suitability for appointment.

However, this matter remained unresolved by the end of the meeting – the first severe test of the Steering Group's authority and also that of its Chair. It did not feel like our finest hour! More discussion was planned to take place before the next meeting, between a local South Birmingham service psychiatrist and myself.

Relations between Henderson Hospital/St Helier NHS Trust and South Birmingham were strained. Henderson's Project Manager wrote to their Director of Planning to reiterate that there was no additional money for refurbishment. This missive followed a telephone call, presumably to the same effect, that had taken place only a fortnight after the Steering Group where this position already had been made abundantly clear. Without doubt some of us involved in this business to replicate the existing Henderson service were more ignorant than others. I, for example, had never before involved myself with the minutiae of NHS funding. I had been blissfully unaware of the important NHS distinction between 'capital' and 'revenue'. While I could grasp the difference once explained (and would thereafter display such erudition to any who would listen), I had not anticipated any difficulty with converting one sort of money into the other, particularly revenue into 'one-off' capital. I did not appreciate that the fiscal crime of turning revenue to capital actually was a capital offence! Nobody had talked about 'capital' for this project, except in connection with the Public–Private Finance Initiative, and then only to dismiss it. At this time (March 1998) no NHS party had successfully emerged from a completed project funded on such a basis. Also our initial time-scale of three years would have been too short to consider such an approach, so the matter had never been progressed. For me this had meant that the capital funding would somehow take care of itself. How wrong I was!

I am not sure now, however, if others in the project shared my naïveté. Perhaps there was a hope, if not expectation, by South Birmingham that capital money could be squeezed out of NSCAG (though they had none) or via their influence on others. Henderson did not, however, share this view and a second battle line was beginning to be drawn between Henderson and South Birmingham. Salford, wisely or cunningly, tended to take a reflective back seat – an apparently concerned observer – in these deliberations. One effect of this was to reinforce a 'good' and 'bad' impression – MHSS appeared much easier to do business with and less ambivalent about the replication enterprise (so was 'good') than did South Birmingham (which was 'bad'). The latter seemed to Henderson to be unable to take up our offers of help, for example, via the Project Manager, who repeatedly reiterated his willingness to assist them with 'funding and viewing relevant buildings and other issues related to the development'.

Interestingly, in the May 1998 Steering Group, a correction was made to the minutes relating to the Consultant appointment, to read as follows: 'The Steering Group agreed that the post of Director should be appointed in line with procedures outlined in the national guidelines for NHS Consultant appointments. It was also agreed that this matter should be discussed further outside the Steering Group before the next meeting.' I cannot now recall the tone of this subsequent discussion nor whether the original minute reflected accurately what had transpired. It is all water under the bridge now and, at least, a decision had been made and the Steering Group was still intact, as the existence of May 1998 minutes testifies.

South Birmingham had identified potential premises near Birmingham, which had been visited, including by Henderson residents – further service-user input and a welcome marker of democratic TC ideology from South Birmingham! This had been an exciting trip in which to take part, and apparently not un-therapeutic for the residents. The coach journey, however, was long, and its tedium only partially relieved by the crunching and sucking of an enormous amount of confectionery purchased at a motorway shop. (We were at this stage unused to subsistence allowances! Receipts, however, had been duly obtained and subsequently submitted to the relevant Trust authorities.) At this stage not much money had reached South Birmingham or Salford and so they were understandably concerned and exercised by any 'risk' associated with committing resources to a project that might be time-limited and last only three years. The Steering Group agreed that the three Chief Executives 'might usefully communicate with one another over this crucial issue'. The costings, including refurbishment costs for South Birmingham, meant that we were potentially in deficit for 1998/99 – an issue that was starting to become a headache. Also, appointing social workers to both of the new services was proving problematic, and negotiations with relevant departments were necessary before any job descriptions could be agreed or posts advertised – another pain!

Decisions, decisions

There is a minute of that 13 May 1998 meeting regarding decision-making. In the meeting we had attempted to discuss the nature of the relationship between the three participating Trusts, NSCAG and the Steering Group, agreeing it to be desirable to define where particular decisions could and should be made (and where not). It was agreed that the Steering Group was the main decision-making forum currently because of the focus on obtaining suitable premises and appointing core senior staff. While premises were being obtained and until the core staff were appointed, the primary financial responsibility would be held by St Helier NHS Trust and managed by the Steering Group. (In this latter forum it was also agreed the three Trusts would negotiate respective budgets and, once set, work within those limits.)

It is mentioned that the Steering Group was responsible for 'key decisions about the project: premises; core staff; planning schedules and other issues of strategic importance'. The appointment of non-core staff would be the responsibility of the individual Trusts, as would building design and other issues 'where local expertise should lead the decision-making process'. Emphatically, though without great clarity or meaning, it was noted, 'the decision-making process should be led by the imperative of seeking a successful outcome to the national development of the three democratic therapeutic communities'. It was 'all for one and one for all' stuff – not actually shedding any more light on who really had the authority and for what!

It was agreed in May 1998 – our fourth meeting of that forum – that the Steering Group should 'operate on the basis of consensus decision-making'. Usefully, it was also agreed that the Project Manager would draft a document outlining in detail the decision-making process, based on the original proposals made in the bid to NSCAG. So at last we could empower ourselves to make the decision to move on to the next agenda item, which concerned staff recruitment! The Henderson process, whereby candidates for vacant posts visit the Unit and meet with residents, was outlined. There was even the idea of a single – 'one for all' – advert for the (medical) Consultant posts but this gained insufficient support from the meeting. Ideologically correct, the idea did not really make sense, since it was better that the two 'Directors' of the new services were appointed before their 'subordinate' Consultant colleagues, for obvious and understandable reasons.

Another important decision was taken in this meeting, namely, to pool the project money, all of which was channelled through St Helier NHS Trust. Any under-spend from Henderson could thus seamlessly flow into whichever of the other services required it. We still did not know which was 'Service 1' and which 'Service 2', since we had no identified premises at this point. Establishing detailed budget plans was therefore problematic. However, it was anticipated there might be under-spend from a slower than expected recruitment to the expanding Henderson Outreach that might be redirected.

In the promised decision-making document prepared by the Project Manager, it was established that the three individual Trusts were responsible for developing detailed plans for the projects in their respective locations. This would entail identifying and preparing property, seeking planning permission, defining recruitment plans and managing the service once established. Such activities would be 'carried out under the general leadership of the Steering Group and with guidance from Henderson Hospital'. This reads to me now as very amateurish. It probably was. But the minutes reflected much labour to reach agreements, often after protracted discussions. It is to be remembered that the Steering Group comprised essentially three groups of people, attempting to work together on a complex project whose success was not guaranteed. The whole process would be closely studied (by independent researchers) and the 'product', if created at all, might have only a very limited life. We were carrying a high level of financial, as well as other, risks. We were working under a heavy time pressure and were not sure if we could deliver. It felt like hard work. Looking back now, perhaps we also made heavy weather of it.

It was established in the decision-making document that the Steering Group could make 'strategic' decisions (not defined) and would oversee the appointment of core staff. The membership of the Steering Group was defined again. For Henderson Hospital this was Director (clinician – me), the Director of Mental Health within the Trust (Manager), Lead Nurse, Research Psychologist and Project Manager, with the Chief Executive and Medical Director (or their nominated deputies) from the other two Trusts. It was also noted that in the event of no consensus being reached, the Chair 'may make executive decisions on behalf of the St Helier NHS Trust'. Lawyers we were not, nor was this Maastricht-style treaty-making, but we hoped we were getting necessary clarity regarding the distribution of authority. Once the premises were secured and the core local staff in place, so it was agreed, the role of the Steering Group would be reviewed. The expectation was that the three individual Trusts would then assume full executive management of the local services. (I remember feeling anxious about claiming power, as Chair, as if this might destabilise our attempts to be democratic or in some way blight the replication process and our guiding 'democratisation' ideology.)

A letter from South Birmingham's Director of Planning brought more headaches, since the refurbishment costs were still included, with no plans to seek alternative funding. Even with unspent monies from Henderson there would still be a shortfall of over £85,000. The Project Manager again advised South

Birmingham to establish a rental cost that might be affordable and sustainable. However, a further concern arose from Birmingham's plan to recruit staff 12 months ahead of admitting residents. A prior agreement had been to appoint the whole staff team by two months prior to opening residential units. The estimated opening date for the South Birmingham 'replica' service also represented a worrying delay to opening (September 1999). (This new projected opening date was still a year earlier than the actual one was to be!) We felt that Birmingham were not speaking the same language or completely on-side with the Steering Group structures or the project as a whole. Whether or not this was accurate, it was Henderson's perception.

Meanwhile the Henderson's own development planning, hard for us to prioritise, continued, though not apace. We had experienced delays with recruiting Outreach staff as previously mentioned. The silver lining to this particular cloud was the increasing level of under-spend available to the rest of the project – at this point, increasing from £90,000 to £113,000. 'Mother' Henderson, however, was feeling the pinch of being under-resourced in personnel terms. (We had insufficient new resource to relieve comfortably those committed to working on the project.) Meanwhile, arrangements for obtaining Consultant posts and junior medical cover were proving difficult in Salford. I stressed the desirability of getting the latter issue discussed locally and had been due to have a meeting myself with some medical staff from the North West. They cancelled this with a promise to re-schedule, which never happened.

The notes of the June 1998 Steering Group report the start of the delay to the North West, via its Regional Outpost, obtaining capital money. Meanwhile South Birmingham were suggesting that their refurbishment costs could be viewed as 'revenue money' and met out of allocated NSCAG resources for 1998/99 and 1999/2000 – £495,000 and £745,000 respectively. There was a re-stating of the core role that ethnicity issues should play in this national development, and it was mooted that the Outreach services should lead on this aspect.

The July 1998 Steering Group minutes show that the North West Regional Outpost had requested from Salford a 'business case'. This was for consideration on 17 July, with a decision likely to be made in September, though possibly as soon as August 1998. Meanwhile in South Birmingham it was not clear whether their preferred premises would need a planning application for change of use. A formidable list of other tasks was identified, which needed addressing prior to the admission of the first residents:

- generate job descriptions and information packs
- advertise posts
- gain knowledge of local catchment area
- develop Outreach model
- develop operational policies

- work with architects
- generate referrals
- assess potential residents
- prepare residents
- train staff
- carry out local PR work.

Local plans would be drawn up in the two new services to reflect this task list!

Henderson agreed to calculate the amount of preparatory work required in relation to potential residents, based on its experience. (It was also noted that within Henderson's Outreach, with its new brief, there was much activity re-defining its service, in particular to specify training. It was thought to be useful for all three Outreach teams to meet to discuss matters of mutual interest, and a meeting was scheduled for August 1998.) Henderson would lead on the actual preparatory work with potential residents. August also saw an early indication of difficulties with obtaining local psychiatric cover, not least since there was still no actual location for the new services!

Location, location, location

The lack of a location for the TCs meant that residential staff recruitment was problematic. In spite of this, it was agreed to begin to develop a marketing strategy for the development to alert potential referrers to these planned future PD specialist services. At least the delay on identifying the premises meant that we had time to devote to 'develop an effective response to culture and ethnicity in the Henderson of the North'. A strategy was proposed for implementation, and this was turned into a detailed project development plan. Even more time was to follow! I was writing to Salford in late October 1998 to complain about the delay in hearing about North West funding, as we still had no reply from their Regional Outpost. At this point it looked as if the deal on Birmingham premises was much closer to clinching than that with Salford. If a significant gap were to open up between the timing of availability of the premises, the result would have been to compromise the second and third strands of the research. (Research funding was fixed and could only cover a period of three years – the larger the gap the less contemporaneous, hence less comparable, would be the findings, and the shorter the period of relevant data collection.)

In the Steering Group we were beginning to think the unthinkable, that we might not be able to set up these services at all. We felt impelled to take what was felt to be an enormous risk. We decided therefore that 'it may be important to consider recruiting the service core staff... even before the premises have been identified'. This suggestion was counter to the prior agreement that 'premises' were driving the process – the Steering Group's mantra up to this point.

Recruiting staff without being able to tell them where they would be based would be highly risky. We could not know how difficult it might be to recruit, in any case, especially given the lack of certainty over funding beyond the setting-up period of three years. Added uncertainty about location might mean that no applicants emerged – the worst case possible. Also, this earlier recruitment option would not be cost-neutral, since some form of accommodation would be required for them in addition to their salary costs. This would represent an additional and unplanned expenditure. But at last some good news. The 7 October 1998 Steering Group minutes reveal that NSCAG had responded positively to the previously stated financial concerns of the Regional Outpost. However, the latter had still not responded to the submitted business case from Salford. Disappointment and annoyance with this lack of decision-making provoked a letter from the Steering Group to NSCAG, to see if they might be able to mediate or intervene to speed up the decision-making process, since we had been led to believe we might have heard in September 1998.

Our letter to NSCAG went from me as Chair and on behalf of the three Chief Executives. However, this process revealed an unexpected grey area. It was not clear whether in fact I could write on their behalf, even though they were notionally members of the Group – they had always been represented by deputies, although circulated with the relevant minutes. The question raised was whether they really had delegated their authority to those attending the Steering Group as their deputies. In practice, at least at times, it appeared that they had not. This meant that some 'decisions' made at Steering Group meetings merely had the superficial appearance of decisions. Local discussion with the Chief Executives would need to take place – necessitating further delay, reflecting the fact that our project, which initially held a reasonably high profile among the Chief Executives, had gradually sunk lower – a factor further exacerbated by changes in their own ranks.

Staff appointments... and premises

Ahead of any identified premises we were to recruit to the Director posts. The Lead Consultant post in Birmingham would be advertised with a corporate style, i.e. including three Trust logos. The Clinical Nurse Manager (Lead Nurse) job description was also in preparation. The interview for the Organisational Researcher – the first strand of the national replication research project – was scheduled for 8 October and it was hoped, given the high quality of the candidates applying, to make an appointment. A pilot study to help identify research measures for the clinical progress strand – researcher to be appointed – was also noted to be under way, under the direction of Dr Chris Evans.

We were now nail-bitingly close to hearing from the North West Regional Outpost: their decisive meeting was due the day following the 11 November Steering Group. So we would all have to wait at least another day. South Birmingham were also waiting, for the result of the NHS strand of competitive tendering for the refurbishment project of their identified premises. The estimated cost of this had increased further to just under £2 million (exclusive of VAT). The good news, so the meeting was told, was that 'planning application was likely' to be successful. That was about as close as we got in that Steering Group meeting to hearing good news about anything.

In case of disappointment, a reserve building had been identified by South Birmingham and it was agreed to provide estimates for its refurbishment also, in the event of the Forhill House option falling through, for whatever reason. I would visit this 'Longbridge' site with local personnel on 23 November. In fact, this site was none other than the Northfield site, famed in TC annals. At the time we had thought this to be auspicious. With all this uncertainty we needed some good omens! It was hard to plan how to spend the available monies, and which amount to apportion to which new service, given that neither service had secured its premises. The Steering Group's request that each of the local services should 'provide an accurate cash flow for 1998/99' now reads as an entirely unreasonable demand.

The deadline for the North West Regional Outpost – 12 November – came and went. Fortunately, none in the Steering Group had been holding their breath. We carried on with our heads, just about, above water! Things were not looking promising, though. However, 'a positive decision was now expected on 11th December 1998' – a potential early Christmas present. 'Agents' had been hired to search for suitable premises in the North West – this sounded exciting and not a little mysterious. But where had all the premises gone? In South Birmingham, an option appraisal between Forhill House and the Longbridge premises was circulated. The Steering Group opted for the latter. It was also agreed that Henderson residents would be asked to ratify this decision – a risky strategy! However, it was agreed, in any case, that design work on Longbridge should commence – so much for residents' verification. There was also a need to identify Outreach service premises for the two new services – more premises to find. And at Henderson we were also drawing up specifications to modify some accommodation for our Outreach team. This, like that previously identified, would come to nothing.

On 11 December we heard, via telephone, that we had got the money for the North West project. We also heard from NSCAG who agreed to meet us (late February/early March) 'with a view to offering positive support' – so says a hand-written note from the Project Manager to me, dated 11 December 1998. The Lead Consultant adverts for South Birmingham and Salford were both placed, and yet more spreadsheets detailing revised development plans were issued. By the 13 January 1999 meeting, Dr Jan Birtle had been appointed to the

South Birmingham Lead Consultant post and Sue Ormrod, the organisational re-searcher, was present to witness this as an 'observer'. The minutes record that the former was warmly congratulated and the latter welcomed. An important corner had been turned, albeit with significant financial risks taken.

Henderson Hospital residents did indeed visit Longbridge and Forhill House, and fortunately the former was preferred. The next Steering Group meeting did thus formally agree that Longbridge was the site for the West Midlands PD service development. The following programme was identified:

- out to tender – March 1999

- back from tender – April 1999

- commence on site – May 1999

- ready for occupation – December 1999 (i.e. almost a year before opening).

The likely cost of the project was £1.4 million, not including VAT! There is also a note, as if the process were not already complicated enough, indicating that the Outreach model adopted by the respective services might affect the type, and possibly size, of the accommodation required. Aaaagh!

South Birmingham were drawing up plans to recruit a Service Manager, as one of the 'core team'. Their idea was to have a time-limited appointment, to be reviewed once the service was fully operational. (This post would not materialise properly for years and would be a source of ongoing stress for those core professionals who were appointed – especially the Lead Consultant and Lead Nurse.) In the North West, a member of the Outreach team would be recruited in Phase 1, along with Lead Consultant, Clinical Nurse Manager, Service Manager, Research Psychologist and administrative support. (Phase 2 would see the recruitment of the remainder of Outreach, and Phase 3 two G grade Charge Nurses and two Social Therapists. The final phase would be to recruit the remainder of the staff team.) South Birmingham also announced that they were in a position to appoint to a specialist registrar post, having secured the required 'national training number' – very good news.

The 10 February 1999 Steering Group meeting was anticipating the meeting with NSCAG on 5 March, and a document for presentation was being prepared by the Project Manager and myself. It would cover:

- introduction/background

- update for South Birmingham, Salford and Sutton

- the training document – from HDT

- future milestones

- budgets

- developmental processes.

An agreed format was adopted by the three Trusts to bring a corporate style to the document. The meeting required drafts of the respective documents for the NSCAG meeting by 19th February – we were taking this meeting with our commissioners very seriously – so that the final document could be circulated on 26 February 1999, i.e. ahead of the scheduled meeting. We were keen to create a favourable impression to mark the success of the partnership to date, notwithstanding it had been a struggle.

Meanwhile, plans were afoot to visit the Longbridge (Northfield) site, with Henderson residents. The South Birmingham Clinical Nurse Manager post job description was all but finalised and the structure of the interview, to include a visit to the Henderson, had also been agreed. Henderson's Lead Nurse would be on the panel. The Salford Director interview was to take place on 19 February 1999, with two representatives from Henderson – a Charge Nurse and myself. A lot seemed to get agreed in this meeting and the minutes were also shorter than usual. Because of a visit to a Dutch TC whilst attending a conference in Amsterdam I had been absent from this Steering Group. Perhaps I should have missed more such meetings! Dr Keith Hyde was appointed to the Salford Director post, as a 'congratulations' letter from me to him attests – more good news. But then we heard that NSCAG had cancelled their meeting with us.

Keith Hyde was formally congratulated on his appointment by the Steering Group in the 10 March 1999 meeting, which happened to be held in Salford, though not in his honour. The permission for the Organisational Researcher to 'track the recruitment process' was beginning its bumpy ride. 'Ethical' objections had been raised, since application forms were considered to be confidential documents, and also because having an observer present might add to the stress of the interview situation. Although this objection was reasonable, it was experienced as an unwelcome impediment to the research process that all parties had accepted as being integral to the original deal. Maybe we felt uncomfortable being observed and powerless to object to the research methodology employed by the independent researchers. The discomfort seemed greatest in Birmingham, serving to open up an old wound. The researcher agreed to seek advice from her supervisor (Professor Ewan Ferlie of Imperial College Management School, London) and helpfully did draw up a statement about the research for the edification of the Steering Group. It was agreed, however, since some important discussions took place outside of the formal meeting arena, that such data were also legitimately part of the organisational research enterprise. It was this agreed that the research did have access to interview 'key individuals' from the three participating Trusts.

As mentioned above, the North West premises were proving problematic and a plan for Henderson Hospital residents to visit their three potential premises did not materialise (for reasons not stated in the March minutes and not now recalled by me). The Project Manager had produced a document – so many of these were generated in the course of this entire project – detailing issues relating to the potential locations. It was only briefly discussed by the Steering Group but my detailed comments, which summarised some of the pertinent issues, at least as I saw them, are reported in full in the following letter:

Dear Keith,

Re: Henderson of the North – implications of where the inpatient unit is sited.

Herewith are my comments on the above document as agreed at the last Steering Group meeting.

I thought that it was extremely useful to put the arguments in such a clear way that allowed for direct comparisons. Clearly not all items listed, for or against, can have equal weighting. I have therefore restricted my comments to those which I feel have most direct impact on the issue of where the inpatient unit might be placed.

Regarding the integration of the unit with existing trusts services, you are obviously far better placed to know the range and variety of existing services but I would imagine that few other trusts in the area could compete with the Salford 'portfolio'. This offers, I would have thought, an unmatched opportunity to integrate the service with others. In particular I would see that educational links with general Psychiatry, Forensic Psychiatry and Psychotherapy could all be very substantial and mutually beneficial. To be sited elsewhere would require an enormous amount of networking which might still deliver a less well and richly integrated service than would be possible with Salford.

Regarding management, the risk of service isolation coupled with large travelling bills (for time and money) are to me overriding considerations which argue strongly in favour of closer siting.

Regarding medical matters, here there would be enormous advantages accruing from having close consultant colleagues offering support for on-call and other matters. The nature of the work stemming from the impact of the personality disordered patients' interpersonal difficulties means that relationships between professional colleagues need to be particularly robust and able to withstand repeated insult! This would be virtually impossible to maintain with colleagues to whom one did not have regular access. The educational aspects of both SHO and Specialist Registrar also argue in favour of going with the local scene given the complex nature of the negotiations and the fact that there may need to be some co-ordination of special hospital, regional secure facility, with the inpatient unit if the specialist registrar is to be trained in Forensic Psychotherapy. (This is my own personal favoured option and I am aware that there is some support for this from Keith and also [X: a local senior clinician].

Regarding staff, there must be overriding advantages of being able to tap the enormous pool of staff potentially available from the 'conurbation'.

I trust that these comments are useful.

With the best wishes.

The pressure was really on us to identify premises since, otherwise, with the lack of progress in South Birmingham we would be unable to operate within the research envelope, when the second and third research strands had begun (see Chapter 6). These needed to collect data from the three sites, and with respect to the two new ones, more or less contemporaneously. It is therefore stated in the minutes that, if we failed to agree on the building by the end of the April 1999 Steering Group meeting, we would need to seek NSCAG's intervention. (What they might have actually said or done in the event we were never to find out.) My own comment on the suitability of Webb House (one of the three identified premises) – requested urgently on 24 March by their newly appointed Director – was that it was 'unsuitable – too institutional, too large/grand and poor location'. The health of the entire replication project looked poor. This was another low point.

In the Steering Group, we stressed the importance of keeping to the agreed time-scale. This required a considerable amount of work, and up to this point we still had only a skeleton staff in each of the two new services who were actually dedicated to the replication task. The Salford Director would have to serve three months' notice and then, for several more months, would still only be able to work half-time on the replication project. With such a scarce resource, no clear funding identified and no premises – meaning no potential to recruit staff wholesale – we felt that we were treading water, already a year into the project. Meanwhile the HDT's training strategy document was presented to the Steering Group and comments invited. Also, recruitment plans for both South Birmingham and Salford were tabled.

At the April 1999 Steering Group meeting, following which the re-scheduled NSCAG meeting would take place (though without resolution of our key financial concern), we held a detailed discussion of the Salford options of premises, taking into account their 'weighted' scores. The latter conveys the thoroughness with which this matter was undertaken. What is missing from the note of that meeting, however, is how much heat the issue under discussion generated. We were constrained by two main factors – cost and speed of delivery. In the end these influenced our decision to opt for a site that, as can be gleaned from my own earlier views, was less than perfect. The minutes record: 'It was agreed that the Steering Group recommended Webb House in Crewe as the preferred option.' This saved us going to NSCAG, although in the event they were coming to us that afternoon in Birmingham!

The meeting with NSCAG turned out to be extraordinarily brief. Although we had had no inkling of it, they had another meeting in a distant part of the country that very afternoon. Given the extent of our preparation and the prior postponement, this was very disappointing. We did not seem to figure highly on NSCAG's list of priorities. A further meeting (between NSCAG and the Project Manager from Henderson), it was decided, would be needed to discuss the financial needs of the project, previously outlined in the letter to NSCAG of 12

March 1999. Although I have no memory of this next point, it was agreed that advice would be given to the new services about the implications of Department of Health guidelines with respect to 'single sex wards'. At least we were always among the first to hear of the latest good idea from the Department of Health. Unfortunately, we were usually also under pressure to conform to it, even if this meant distorting the treatment model we were simultaneously called upon to replicate.

In that same short NSCAG meeting, South Birmingham was admonished for wanting to operate a non-ageist admission policy, i.e. unlike Henderson's (politically incorrect) 18 to 45 age range. NSCAG declared, since the Henderson Hospital model was to be replicated as closely as possible, that the age range must stand. The minutes records a concession that 'some minor variation would be inevitable'– somewhat at variance with other NSCAG advice that 'replication is what the three of you agree it is'. Our 'Project Update' for NSCAG, prepared by us with great care back in February, was to be 'circulated for detailed consideration'.

This meeting with NSCAG had been unsatisfactory. They had been made aware of our financial concerns previously. This major topic, however, had been all but avoided in the perfunctory meeting that took place. No time was given to the project update nor to acknowledging what (albeit limited) progress had been made with the project so far and what were the future milestones and our other plans. It seemed that NSCAG was seriously under-resourced. I was accused over the telephone of 'harassment', when trying to make telephone contact after repeated letters had gone unanswered over a period of weeks. At least the Steering Group's agreement over Webb House as suitable premises had meant that we did not need to burden NSCAG with having to think about us on that score! They had played their decisive role, saying 'yes' to our bid in 1997. Perhaps it was too early in their recovery phase to expect more potency.

The 14 April 1999 Steering Group meeting minutes recall that we were still awaiting approval from NSCAG for the detail of 1999/2000 funding. For established services that have been and will continue to be a secure part of the NHS, not knowing details of funding is not so problematic. Life goes on, albeit often with an effectively smaller budget to spend than for the previous year. However, services not yet established need to know in advance what their financial constraints are. For such financial issues therefore to be summarily discussed, as they were in the meeting with NSCAG, was to my mind insensitive to those of us trying to spend taxpayers' money responsibly. In fact, a letter was sent to us that day detailing April's payments and implying that further discussion was not needed. From our calculations, however, the figures did not add up. We believed there were indeed matters to discuss. Therefore I wrote on behalf of the Steering Group to seek clarification.

Miscellaneous issues

What on the face of it looked like being a dull 'extraordinary' meeting (on a spectacularly sunny day – for Salford – 27 May 1999) proved to be very productive. It was set up to identify the nitty-gritty, detailed activity required to replicate the Henderson both administratively and managerially. Thus we needed 'to establish milestones and outline the process by which a person enters and leaves the service'. On the way, it was hoped that other aims might also be achieved, namely to:

- prioritise the development of elements of the service
- inform development of the operational policy
- identify policies and resources already available
- recognise and define pieces of work each of us can do for ourselves and each other
- inform and define the design and usage of the building.

You had to be dedicated to sit through this sort of stuff. And the Henderson contingent had needed to be in Prestwich (on the far side of Manchester) by 10.30 a.m. that day. Another early morning in Euston railway station.

The May 1999 Steering Group meeting brought good news from the front line on the ethics of recruitment tracking. Sue Ormrod had been given the go-ahead to meet with Directors of Human Resources. All job descriptions would have a 'form of words' to inform prospective candidates of the existence of the research. Meanwhile, we felt we still did not have sufficient clarity regarding finances in order for South Birmingham to progress their premises – they were in the thick of the tendering process at this time (see earlier). It was agreed therefore that we would ask the Director of Finance within the new Trust to seek clarification from NSCAG that sufficient funds were available for 1999/2000. (Note that we were in a different Trust now. The process of merging brought an added source of stressors – for example, five managers of Henderson during a so-called 'steady state year' in which to consolidate the merger.) Without this clarification of finances, we could not progress the premises and without that we could not complete recruitment, hence no new services at all might be the result – so this was an important issue. South Birmingham were understandably anxious and irritated. In the Steering Group, we all were. (Having NSCAG as such a negative presence did help our cohesion as a group – on the odd occasion.)

At this point, we were planning to admit residents in June 2000, even though we still did not know which service would emerge first, hence to where they might be admitted. It was recognised that two new referral bases would need to be developed and prospective residents identified and prepared. To this end, the importance of recruiting Outreach staff, funding permitting, was stressed. Salford had duly circulated an 'Outreach Strategy' document and comments on this were to be sent to their Director. A Lead Nurse for South Birmingham,

Michael Bennett, had been appointed with a planned start date of 14 June. His appointment was warmly welcomed. Some limited recruitment was thus still possible, but no one felt confident in doing this. Recruiting staff under such circumstances was far from ideal. It was also noted that the project needed a unified 'information strategy' for responding to NSCAG, though reasons for this being included at this point are not stated. The lack of unity in this respect, perhaps itself partly a reflection of lack of local management support, would prove to be part of our ultimate undoing.

The 27 May 1999 meeting had been helpful in identifying the limits of our mutual understanding of, for example, the role of Outreach. The South Birmingham Director developed this in a letter of 15 June. In particular she identified 'the importance of allowing the team to develop and in the end to have some parameters within which they can be boundaried'. This recognises the needs, perhaps inherent in all new teams, to be able to have a say in the direction and pace of their own development. In contrast to the residential aspect of this replication project, the Outreach staff had permission to become more truly themselves.

The Project Manager (from Henderson) had spoken to the NSCAG Secretary on the phone on 3 June, about refurbishment expenditure, after he had made many fruitless calls – a note from the Project Manager states as much. The telephone call was followed by a letter from the secretary. Incidentally it illustrated something of the relationship between the centre (commissioning) and the periphery (the three Trusts). The 'centre' showed little sign of urgency in relation to decisions being made.

Given the obstacles to be overcome by those developing these new services, this attitude, from the 'periphery' was unhelpful. There was an assumption that the South Birmingham Trust had not questioned the refurbishment costs nor its capital allocation. The Chief Executive and Medical Director of the Trust were, in effect, full members of the Steering Group, or at least in touch with their deputies, hence such matters would certainly have been considered. It would seem that the Trust, however, might not have explored fully the situation with their relevant Regional Office, although equally well they may have been aware that no capital was available from that source – the NHS after all was not awash with capital. There is an acknowledgement of the problem incurred, however, as well as directions in which to take things further. But why were these not stated back in February? My letter to Dr 'Z' (dated 14 June) conveys some of the frustration felt by those of us in the Steering Group.

Dear [Z],

Re: Severe Personality Disorder – nationwide service development.

I enclose the draft document, which outlines the background to the present impasse to the above development, and, in particular, that relating to the premises, which the Steering Group has been working to secure for the service based in South Birmingham. This document will form part of a larger one used in the negotiation with West Midlands Regional Office.

As you know, I have explained the implications of the delay in agreeing 1999/2000 funding on the overall service development and, as importantly, the negative impact on the independent assessment exercise. The Steering Group will therefore need to consider at its meeting in July whether or not a formal complaint about the lack of constructive support for this development from the Department will need to be lodged.

Please could you give me the necessary information as to how to lodge such a complaint and with whom? You will see that I will be copying this letter to [Secretary to NSCAG], Professor [B: Chair of Steering Group – Research] and Professor [C: co-investigator].

Yours sincerely.

Dr Z's reply displayed the elegant (circular) simplicity of the civil servant system. To complain formally about X one needs to write to X! The 'three' of us could be united in the face of NSCAG. But, back at the 9 June Steering Group, we were amending the minute referring to the agreement to select Webb House to reflect South Birmingham's 'reservations...about the location in relation to the Birmingham service' and to stake the territorial claim that 'all of the West Midlands region would be served by them'. Did the three participating Trusts truly trust one another? In any event, the meeting distilled a number of issues from the previously mentioned, sunny and successful 27 May meeting, as follows:

- the need for an Outreach strategy for the period prior to the TC opening (assessment and preparation) and for when the service was open and fully operational

- the need for clear training for the Outreach team before starting the preparatory work with prospective residents

- the need for secretarial and administrative staff to be effectively trained

- the need to develop links with referrers, so as to produce 'informed' referrals

- the need to define the interaction between Outreach and the in-patient therapeutic community.

We noted that the agreed monthly sum for March 1999 was being paid, but this monthly amount, for the whole year, did not provide a sufficient total figure for the development. In an attempt to improve communication between the Steering Group, Regional Offices and NSCAG, it was agreed to invite NSCAG to quarterly review meetings to discuss finances, activity and progress against milestones. This felt like the tail (Steering Group) wagging the dog (NSCAG). As if to add further

pressure, South Birmingham informed the Steering Group that the most acceptable tender received by them was only valid for a period of three months. After
this the whole tendering process might need to be repeated, with the likelihood
that returned tenders would be higher than those currently on the table. Also, a
potential building for Outreach services in Birmingham had been identified but it
was in need of some refurbishment…!

With puzzlement we heard that South Birmingham had insufficient funds to
appoint a Business Manager – was this a false economy or a chess move in the
game with NSCAG (and with 'us')? Henderson pointed out that there was money
identified in the original bid for such a post. The idea of a secondment to the
managerial post was raised. What exactly was going on? Surely it would have
helped all concerned to have somebody taking on this crucial management role in
South Birmingham. The (relative) 'good guys' in Salford were advertising, among
others, for their Business Manager. Indeed, with no money having changed
hands, the *Crewe Guardian* had got wind of the premises business and billed our
project as front-page news. It read: 'New home for the disturbed: mental health
service plans change of use for Webb House'. We had not reckoned on the fact
that this former orphanage held such a pride of place in local hearts, even with its
having been a British Rail property most recently. It might have been that the
prospect of Salford's 'disturbed' coming to reside locally caused the Crewe folk
to reassess the value of local properties, including their own homes.

A crucial meeting with NSCAG and the Regional Office about the funding
of the South Birmingham premises had taken place on 9 July 1999. It had been
constructive, and a letter from NSCAG confirming what had been agreed was
eagerly awaited. (This duly arrived on 16 July.) The South Birmingham Trust
Board were meeting on 21 July, when it was hoped a decision to proceed with
'Longbridge' would be made. It was noted that NSCAG had requested that
capital charges were re-examined and that set-up costs should be recorded separately from the ongoing service provision costs. The Steering Group thanked
those South Birmingham staff who had prepared the relevant documentation for
this important meeting. It represented, perhaps, a turning point for us in our
being more mature and confident and able to be more conciliatory and less
paranoid towards NSCAG. To prevent any such recurrence of this set of difficulties it was decided to set up four monthly meetings with the mental health leads
from the NHS regional offices, although these never materialised. Perhaps they
represented 'a meeting too far'.

It was now revealed that, even once agreed, the work on the South Birmingham premises would still take 40 weeks. The summer months, when building
work progresses more swiftly, had been lost. This would cause delay to the
planned opening. Contrary to the 'hopeful' headline of the *Crewe Guardian*, and
much to our collaborative relief, a 'change of use' was not required for Webb
House and negotiations were now under way to purchase the building. The Organisational Researcher protocol for interviewees was still progressing – slowly.

The November 1999 Steering Group minutes recall that Henderson Hospital's own search for Outreach premises was again coming to nothing. As a marker of the seriousness of the situation, our Chief Executive had been informed of this, in writing. Also, as Steering Group Chair, I had written to the Chief Executive of the Mental Health Services of Salford with respect to delays in the North West. Completion of purchase of Webb House was expected to be November 1999, and the tendering process for refurbishment had at last begun. In South Birmingham refurbishment work had actually started, with the planned opening in June 2000. Planning permission for Hendersons' Outreach premises was also expected this month (November 1999).

A good response had been obtained to the Consultant post (Outreach/ residential) advertisement in Salford but none to that from South Birmingham. The three of us Directors would meet to discuss this further. The 'shift system' put in an effort to become the most problematic and divisive issue within the Steering Group, now that we had resolution on so many other financial and building-related matters! (After that we would have the issue of 'IT' with which to run and run, in case we got complacent.) A correction to the October meeting minutes reads as follows: 'resentment' should read 'recruitment'. What was going on in our unconscious minds?

A site visit to the Birmingham premises was planned for 12 January 2000. In case that sounded a too positive note, a new question had been raised about the need for ethical approval for the organisational research, although the clear view of the Chair of its Supervisory Group held that this was not at all necessary. (This necessitated a lengthy but ultimately fruitless exercise in identifying and contacting the relevant local Research Ethics Committees.) Successes and failures with recruitment were noted. Included in this was a discussion of how to ensure a 'culturally diverse' team. Contracts had been exchanged for Webb House – precise opening dates now stood at 11 February 2000 for Outreach and 24 July for the residential unit. Our own South London/Central London hunt for Outreach premises was less successful. The national service's marketing material, however, was ready to go to the printers. Lots of activity and not a little progress.

Catchment, recruitment and shift patterns

With the issue of premises being at least partially sorted, there still remained formidable obstacles to be overcome before the residential units could open. Principal among these was that of staff recruitment. However, there were other issues that emerged as problematic – agreement over the catchment areas of the three services, details of the shift pattern in relation to replication and on-call cover. And still there were issues unresolved with respect to the Organisational Researcher and her access to the services under study, which was exasperating!

Discussion at the 9 February 2000 Steering Group had touched on the issue of catchment areas but without definitive conclusion having been reached. There was thus an ongoing correspondence about this matter, which would stretch into spring 2000. Part of this centred on sensitivity to the existing area of Francis Dixon Lodge, a long-established democratic therapeutic community in Leicester. We all wanted to maintain good relations with our colleagues there. The other sensitive issue, however, was that to do with the proximity of our two new services and a suspicion of unhelpful rivalry between the West Midlands and North West services. At this point another potential rival arrived! This was a Salford-inspired course on 'Systems-Centred Therapy' – due to take place on 4 and 5 July 2000. The rivalry here was of another kind – a different approach to group-work from that operated at Henderson (group-analytic). The ostensible idea was that this approach could 'inform Webb House staff how the different groups and activities within the Unit interrelate'. This perhaps represented a subtle undermining of the democratic TC by Salford, even though this new staff team incorporated three ex-Henderson staff.

Early March 2000, however, saw the start of a healthy stream of staff recruited to the South Birmingham and Salford ranks. In Birmingham, for example, the Director, Lead Nurse, Project Officer, two Adult Psychotherapists, Principal Social Therapist, two Senior Nurse Therapists, four Nurse Therapists, PA to Director, receptionist and temporary clerical support were all in post. Three candidates were due to be interviewed for a Consultant Psychiatrist/Psychotherapist post on 9 March, having attended a viewing day in Henderson on 2 March. Applications had been received for further Senior Nurse and Nurse Therapist posts, for two Senior Social Therapists, Senior Creative Therapist, Research Assistant, Research Fellow and Lecturer Practitioner. Some of these would be the fodder for the 5 x 2 days course due to start in Birmingham on 1 May 2000 (see Chapter 2).

In Salford, the news was also good, although recruitment lagged behind that of South Birmingham. Posts were at the later stages of finalisation and going out to advert. Meanwhile at Henderson three staff had been recruited to fill vacancies – two Social Therapists and a Nurse. The rotating junior doctor had been persuaded to stay on for a further six months to 'provide continuity', an indirect statement that (with the high turnover of staff) this had been difficult to maintain adequately. Further Henderson posts were due to be interviewed – two 'H' grade Nurses – one in the residential and one in the Outreach – a locum Clinical Psychologist and a Researcher. One member of staff was on maternity leave, with two about to go on it, in the spring. But one had returned from maternity leave, so that gave reason for encouragement. One staff member was noted to be on 'long-term sick leave' but another was returning from the same. Lots of swings, lots of roundabouts!

Importantly, there had been an extraordinary meeting to discuss replication on 1 March 2000. It had been this meeting where the idea to form a Replication Meeting had been hatched (see Chapter 4). In particular, there was the issue of replicating Henderson's shift pattern, which exercised all concerned. The extent to which this became an issue can be seen from the fact that the matter had been referred to the South Birmingham Trust's solicitor and a very lengthy response had been received – not appended here.

Bad news travels fast

As if to counter March's good news on the recruitment front, there was adverse press publicity in response to the proposed siting of the Crewe-based service. Gloomily a report in a local newspaper noted that the completion of the project was contrary to the wishes of the community and that despite reassurance from the clinical director of the Trust, local people were still worried about the ramifications of having a residential unit in the area and the possibility that many patients would express their problems through threatening behaviour, whether to themselves or others. The piece concluded on an 'upbeat' note, mentioning that the refurbishment of the building would at least secure its future – implying that the fabric of the building appeared to be of greater importance than its human contents!

The April 2000 Steering Group meeting brought good news, in that 'brokerage arrangements' between our Trust and NSCAG had been successfully agreed. Thanks were to be relayed to our Director of Finance, Peter Cardell. For each piece of good new, however, there seemed to be at least one of bad. Salford reported that no application to the part-time Consultant Psychotherapist post had been received. It was already in business, however, with 51 referrals having been accepted (by 11 March). So was South Birmingham, which had received 40 referrals, having only opened its doors on 1 March.

By the time of the 16 June 2000 monthly Steering Group meeting, South Birmingham had appointed 34 staff, although certain key posts remained unfilled – part-time Consultant, two Clinical Psychologists and various secretarial vacancies. Salford, still lagging behind on recruitment, had plans on how to open the residential unit and the complementary roles that Outreach and residential staff would occupy in relation to this task. Meanwhile, at Henderson the vacant senior nurse post was in the process of being filled. That month also saw the Association of Therapeutic Communities (ATC) experiential weekend – expertly provided for us by Rex Haigh and Jean Rees. The Systems-Centred Therapy experiential workshop (directed by two eminent Americans, Fran Carter and Susan Gantt) was also scheduled.

The 14 July Steering Group and Replication Meetings were cancelled but an Annual Report (1999–2000), compiled by the three services for NSCAG, provides an important summary of the project up to July 2000. Among other aspects, it describes the prominent role of HDT (and especially that of the Volunteers) in the recruitment of staff. Thus HDT is reported as collaborating with the local team in South Birmingham to design and implement 'selection days'. Initially these were staged at Henderson but later at Bridger House (Outreach headquarters in Birmingham), the change of venue and structure being developed in response to the need to meet the required time-scale for recruitment. The involvement of ex-residents was said to have been '*in monitoring candidates' attitudes to meaningful user participation, a central part of the service philosophy*'. South Birmingham were strongly embracing Henderson's collaborative TC ideology by this stage in the project.

A similar range of activities to that in South Birmingham was under way in Crewe. The Salford Mental Health Services contribution to the Annual Report details the delay in the opening, as well as some of the reasons for this. It comments that 'major issues about replication have been worked through, including staff mix, the programme, the "rules" protocols and policies, and the shift system'. As with South Birmingham, Volunteers were acknowledged to be closely involved in 'psycho-education' and selection of new residents. The first meeting with potential residents happened on 30 April in Gaskell House in central Manchester, with alternating weekly introductory meetings and selection groups. The input from HDT staff and Volunteers to the selection of residents was agreed to continue on a weekly basis, but only up until four weeks post-opening (a letter from the Project Manager dated 25 August refers). In this letter, the Project Manager's resignation and imminent leaving were mentioned. This was to represent a significant loss to the project. Effective communication would be one early and obvious casualty.

There is a brief but interesting report, written by local staff, documenting a meeting between members of HDT – staff and Volunteers – and South Birmingham staff, focusing on the latter's therapeutic programmes. While emphasising that the 'core groups' would remain the same as Henderson's, the meeting was to focus on possible differences between the two. Regarding the shift system, HDT, apparently, 'expressed concern about (dis) continuity of staff presence in the evenings/ night'. The proposed 'end of day community meeting' in South Birmingham was thought to be either too stimulating or preventing closure! Volunteers thought that it would get in the way of the evening 'recovery' from the intensity of the day. The Saturday morning presence of medical staff was argued to be important for both practical medical and (symbolic) emotional support – for staff as well as residents. Modifications to the programme in relation to starting up were also considered. These concerned the possibility of starting solely with 'practically-based groups to do with living tasks', adding in the rest of the programme only later. There seemed to be an HDT concern that moving into the full programme later might prove problematic.

The Units opened on 12 September (Webb House) and 19 September (Main House). South Birmingham's plan, after discussion with HDT, was to start with a cohort of 16 residents and slowly build to its maximum of 27. At the time of opening the Birmingham service had received 101 referrals from which an 18-strong cohort was selected. These had all completed information sessions, pre-selection and selection – the latter sessions being chaired by the Volunteers.

The selected residents had also cooked their first meal in Main House on 7 September. The staff induction to Main House had included a 24-hour 'experiential event', facilitated by ATC on 1–2 September to aid orientation to the building. (Six posts, however, including the Consultant Psychotherapist (part-time post), remained unfilled.)

There is a note in the Steering Group minutes of 13 September, held in Birmingham, that Webb House had opened successfully the day before, in spite of an ugly protest by local people, which had threatened to mar the occasion. A celebratory meal, was planned for Friday 15 September to mark the end of the first week's programme. This was an anxious time, not relieved by the knowledge that in Birmingham, during their first week of operation, all three emergency services had been involved in the course of a single night! Mercifully, the reasons did not reflect the feared outbreak of pandemonium – fire alarms had been triggered falsely, one resident had an acute physical illness (necessitating an ambulance trip to the local A&E department) and somebody was attempting to break into the Unit, so staff had called the police!

Occupation of Webb House saw a still incompletely refurbished building. It was 12 days before heating, hot water and kitchen equipment were functioning satisfactorily. There was no computer network and the residents' pay phones had not been installed. (The national fuel shortage which coincided had not helped matters.) As with Main House, staff had occupied the building prior to opening with residents, spending the night of 7 September there, increasing staff confidence in 'managing the building'. Eleven residents had been admitted on 12 September, plus four in late September and a further four in early October. A 'community of 13' was said to be 'continuing to function' by 11 October, the time of the next Steering Group. The programme was claimed to be 'remarkably similar to that of Henderson'. The importance of clearly defining therapy groups, to reduce the pressure for all meetings to be 'therapy', was recognised by Webb House staff. Sadly, it was clear that some staff and residents had been, and others felt, physically threatened by some of the Crewe locals.

The headlines, some front page – 'Webb House War of Words' (*Crewe Chronicle*, 25 October 2000), 'Assurance over unit is insufficient: angry residents [local people] storm out of public meeting' – reveal what a tempest our occupation of Webb House had indeed stirred up. However, this was fuelled in part by local party politics. Two sides were represented. 'Labour' was accused of having branded the Unit's local opponents as 'bigots'. Less extreme views were also to be found on the topic on the inside pages of the local newspapers, for example, under the headline 'Those we know pose a danger', a letter from a local person made the thoughtful point that 'threats to...well-being [do not] come from demonised strangers...[but] from people we know'. Although this was not front-page news, it was still welcome (*Crewe Chronicle*, 20 September 2000).

Conclusions

The long wait for confirmation of the success of the bid to NSCAG no doubt caused some loss of momentum. This time delay meant changes to the staff who had been involved in the original bid. Consequently, much of the early excitement about and prioritising of the replication project was lost, as it became eclipsed or submerged by other Trust matters. But it was possible to rekindle the flame of enthusiasm. The fact that the groundwork was begun without central financing is a testament to the real investment of the Trusts involved. However, the extent to which resources could be dedicated ahead of funding was necessarily limited. The fact that the delivery of the full financing was delayed added to difficulties, albeit offering us more time to finalise detailed plans.

The problems encountered with capital funding were frustrations that we could all have done without and, not surprisingly, the anxiety associated with identifying capital expenditure had a negative effect on the collaboration. All of us became more anxious, since at times it looked as if the whole project might founder on account of difficulties surrounding this. As the time taken to identify premises (in all three services) and associated developments mounted, it became easy for Henderson to see its partners as partially to blame and, compared to ourselves, only partially invested in the project. The agreed initial strategy not to appoint staff until the premises had been identified, although probably correct, had the effect of locating the project's administrative and strategic burden disproportionately on Henderson. Until the appointment of the Directors of the two embryonic services, there were no exactly equivalent positions from which to champion the development in the other two Trusts. Fortunately, two 'local champions' were appointed and they helped to propel matters.

Overall, although there was considerable (18 months) slippage from the original plan, the Steering Group had developed into a cohesive unit and delivered a complex project almost within budget. The original plan for its role and the other managerial structures envisaged, especially that of the HDT, appeared to be at least adequate to the task. We had moved, from being relative strangers and naïve with respect to an innovative project of large size and complexity, to being professionals who could confront at least some difficulties and resolve disagreements with determination and (relative) patience – at least on a good day. Indirectly, NSCAG had aided our cohesion as a group, through occupying the (not entirely deserved) role of common enemy.

Part III

Reviewing the Project

CHAPTER SIX

The Proof of the Pudding

Introduction

Evaluating the Henderson replication experiment was an integral aspect of this project, since it had been mandated by the commissioners of the service – NSCAG. For reasons of probity it would need to be shown whether replication had been achieved. If so, then it might be that central funding would continue. If not, there would be no central funding, hence no national severe personality disorder service. The research aspect was integral to the bid to NSCAG and, with the help of DH personnel, it had been part of Henderson's original submission to them. Thus we had reason to believe that we had also secured relevant Department of Health funding for the submitted research methodology. Others, independent of Henderson and the other two Trusts, would carry out this research evaluation in due course. Without a funded research project our bid would have been incomplete, hence uncompetitive.

The research aspect of the bid was generated mainly by the Henderson researcher, Fiona Warren, and myself, with advice and support from Professor Nick Black and Dr Nick Graves (London School of Hygiene and Tropical Medicine) and Dr Dilys Jones and Dr Sheila Adam (Department of Health/Home Office). It included a broad outline of a three-stranded method, one qualitative and two quantitative strands: organisational; clinical; and health economic. The detailed methodology would be provided by those supervising and undertaking the actual research, once the success of the bid to NSCAG had been guaranteed. No one external to the bid had been prepared to undertake detailed work until the bid for replication had proved to be successful. At the time, there was no national severe personality disorder service to research. There was no guarantee that any such service would ever exist. In the event, ours was one of only three (out of 57) successful bids submitted to NSCAG that year to receive funding.

It was the then High Security Psychiatric Services Commissioning Board that, we believed, had agreed to fund the research – in the region of £500,000. Unfortunately for us, the delay in the decision of NSCAG to endorse the bid (see Chapter 1) meant that this grant-giving body was itself changing. One tiresome result of this was an extremely exhausting set of meetings with them, over many months. During this time, the original grounds for undertaking the research appeared to be ignored by the new personnel who were established to oversee such grants. These new personnel demanded a randomised controlled trial of democratic therapeutic community treatment outcome (versus treatment as usual). They appeared to ignore the basic requirement of NSCAG, which was for the research project to be an evaluation of the *replication* exercise.

Valiantly, but for a long time vainly, Fiona Warren and I battled to represent the originally agreed replication brief for the project. However, the ears upon which our repeated arguments fell were deaf, and the minds, at best, amnesic. In successive meetings we would apparently succeed in reminding those grant-givers concerned that the *replication* (not effectiveness) brief had been imposed upon us by NSCAG. However, we would discover in each subsequent meeting that we had to re-argue the same point all over again. This was an exasperating state of affairs that caused enormous ill feeling and was only finally resolved contractually with a form of words that committed us to consider randomisation where appropriate. (In fact an NHS R&D-funded feasibility exercise was later undertaken, which suggested, at least to the chair of the body supervising the replication research, that this was not a feasible option.) Unfortunately even this did not end the wrangling. Eventually the head of the National Research and Development Programme became involved and these matters were finally settled. This represented a chapter in the Henderson replication story best left untold. It will not be further reported here.

Happily, strong research collaborations were established between Imperial College Management School, London (organisational strand), St George's, University of London (clinical progress strand) and the London School of Hygiene and Tropical Medicine (health economic strand). These enabled the research to start, albeit slightly delayed, under the overall supervision of a group chaired by Professor Nick Black, already referred to above. The three research strands reported regularly to this forum (as well as to the funders) in order to guarantee fidelity to the research brief and the independence of the research exercise from the clinical replication project.

Unfortunately, not everything was plain sailing. Early on there were difficulties with identifying the necessary ethical approval apparatus and with gaining access to the relevant parts of the services (see also Chapter 5), which looked like jeopardising the work of the organisational strand. Later on, the loss of the in-house research support in the three services, occasioned by NSCAG's withdrawal of funding from these posts, threatened the second and third strands' success – a last-ditch attempt by NSCAG to de-rail the work they had mandated? Also, a request to fund some extra research to integrate the results of all three strands of this work (that might have brought considerable added value to an under-researched area in the field) was turned down by our funders. As there had already been an extension to our funding, this was not altogether surprising, but nevertheless disappointing.

All the eventual (independent) researchers involved in this project are to be congratulated on their commitment to the task and their resilience in the face of obstacles encountered – most notably the three Research Fellows, Dr Sue

Ormrod (organisational), Dr Matthew Fiander (clinical progress) and Dr Sue Langham (health economic). They were supervised by Professors Ewan Ferlie (previously Imperial College Management School, London and now Royal Holloway), Tom Burns (previously St George's, University of London and now Kellogg College, Oxford) and Charles Normand (previously London School of Hygiene and Tropical Medicine and now Kennedy Professor, University College, Dublin).The substance of this chapter derives from my understanding of their work and the final reports submitted by them to the funding authorities – Forensic Mental Health R&D (successor to the HSPSCB).

An academic view of replication

UK public policy initiatives stress the need to improve public services through the diffusion of 'evidence-based models' or 'good practice', from small pockets across the wider system (DoH 2001). Agencies such as the former NHS Modernisation Agency try to spread service redesign techniques across the NHS. But it is not established that an innovation – especially of a complex human service, such as Henderson's democratic TC – really can be spread in such a planned way. To do justice to the study of such complex processes, the research field relating to 'organisations' has developed non-linear analyses of innovations. A brief summary of this aspect of the field therefore may be pertinent.

Recognising the fact that innovations tend to be modified or redesigned by the user, i.e. 'reinvention' (Rogers 1983), recent organisational studies emphasise the dynamic nature of the innovation process (Lewis and Seibold 1993), referring to it as one of 'appropriation' as much as dissemination (Clark 1987). Non-linear approaches see innovation processes as being characterised by interactions from many actors in a fluid arena (Van de Ven *et al.* 1999). In much of healthcare, many interacting factors – organisational context, actors and activities (Fitzgerald *et al.* 2002) – shape innovation. The instantiation of an innovation is the result of particular events and coalitions of things and people (networks) gaining meaning. From this perspective, there is no solid 'thing' that gets passed on, rather a process that may be transformative of the innovation itself. On this basis, a policy-maker's notion of 'best practice' may be oversimplified. Organisational forms or systems that work well in one location are not necessarily readily transferable to another context (Robertson, Swan and Newell 1996).

At the start, those of us involved in submitting the bid to NSCAG had considered 'replication' to be a relatively simple matter of 'pass–fail'. Either the Henderson service would be replicated or not. It might have been replicated in one site but not the other. In retrospect, however, 'failure' was probably not the most appropriate concept. It might have been more accurate to construe the issue of replication as dimensional, hence degrees of replication. Dr Ormrod, in her final report, discusses three main obstacles to a simple, categorical 'pass–fail' measure: the 'spirit and letter' problem; the issue of when to sample; and the issue of pluralism, as applied to a multiple stakeholder or complex situation.

Considering the spirit and letter problem in respect of replication, there are four possible interpretations: (1) followed in the spirit; (2) not followed in the spirit; (3) followed to the letter; (4) not followed to the letter. 'Replication' might be assigned to any two of the four categories, by a given observer. This yields four possible verdicts – followed neither in spirit nor to the letter; followed in spirit but not to the letter; followed to the letter but not in spirit; and followed both in spirit and to the letter. The more the 'letter' is only imprecisely specified and/or the 'spirit' allows for alternative interpretations, the more there is room for disagreement among observers. With this replication project there was both an imprecise letter and a permissive spirit, leaving much room for doubt and debate over how replication research results might be interpreted. (This situation posed problems for the implementors (see also Chapters 3 and 4) as well as for the organisational strand researchers.)

The replication of Henderson was neither simple to achieve nor to assess. In the absence of detailed specification plans from the three participating organisations, and in the interests of the organisational research strand, the researcher and her supervisor had needed to operationalise the concept of 'replication'. Four principles were taken to underpin their investigation:

1.   The new organisations need not be exact copies of Henderson, for replication to occur. This is because the Henderson model puts a premium on participatory decision-making and flexible structures so that literal similarities between the new sites and Henderson might even be evidence of non-replication.

2.   Replication requires only that the new sites should be 'Henderson-like', acknowledging that some departures from literal replication may be benign (local adaptations).

3.   Replication must go beyond that of formal structures, since the Henderson model rests fundamentally on work practices, culture and values, some of which are subtle.

4.   There is a need to allow for modernisation of the Henderson model in relation to aspects, such as risk management and the European Working Time Directive.

Applying these four principles, successful replication was to be evidenced by the presence of structures, work practices and underlying values that were 'Henderson-like'.

The fact that this project concerned innovation meant that there was room for debate about when the emergent (new) TCs might be ready to be measured, not only against one another but against the Henderson blueprint. It was not clear at which point any relevant 'sample' (of the TC's structure, practices or culture) should be taken by the organisational researcher (or by the HDT). Taken too early, the sample might be immature for comparative purposes; too late, an unnecessarily lengthy, hence costly, evaluation exercise would have been funded. However, it was not possible to know what was 'just right'. According to Dr Ormrod's report, most respondents thought that five years might be about the right period to have elapsed, but this was not feasible for a variety of reasons. The organisational research coat had to be cut according to its cloth – the period that had originally asked for (three years), plus one year's extension in acknowledgement of the delay in finding premises and opening the residential units.

Evidence from the organisational strand

Research method

Organisational academics suggest that *organising* is more profound than the *organisation*, seen in ongoing and fluctuating work practices amongst organisational members (Czarniawska 1997; Stacey 2000; Weick 1995). An ethnographic approach was therefore adopted in order to explore organisational culture and daily work practices as well as formal structures and procedures (Hatch 1997; Rapoport 1960; Rosen 1991). Ethnography has been widely used in organisational studies (Meek 1988; Rosen 1991), given an appreciation that organisational culture is locally situated and best observed through the study of concrete behaviours. In keeping with the ethnographic orientation (Becker *et al.* 1977), the chosen method was not to test specific hypotheses but to enter the field theoretically sensitised to organisational analysis and with a defined substantive problem.

Dr Ormrod worked across the three geographically dispersed sites (South London, Birmingham and Greater Manchester/Crewe), covering 140 staff and 250 residents over a period of 3.5 years. Her fieldwork covered the service set up over two years (Phase 1) and the first 18 months in the life of the two new therapeutic communities (Phase 2). Four key methods were used: observation; interviews and informal conversation; document collection; and member checking (i.e. presenting researchers' findings to those interviewed/studied with a view to receiving their further feedback – to be amalgamated with earlier findings). Fieldwork was concentrated on the Henderson site in Phase 1 to understand 'the model' but on the two new sites in Phase 2.

In the absence of detailed specifications for developing the service, the major foci in Phase 1 were determinations of what 'the model' was, what replication meant for participants and how it might be meaningfully assessed. As is usual in ethnographic research study design, data collection and early analysis were iterative and developed in the course of research (Hammersley and Atkinson 1995). Fieldwork was based on a broad observation of each TC service as a whole. More concrete foci were developed during later data collection, analysis and writing (Becker *et al.* 1977). For assessing whether the model had been appropriated ('replicated') in the new sites, the final analysis focused on three aspects of structure and procedures as 'tracers' (staffing and organisational profile; structure of the therapeutic programme; the residents' career and its management) and three aspects of day-to-day practice considered to reveal the enactment of organisational culture (flattened hierarchy and take-up of responsibility; staff–resident boundaries and therapeutic engagement).

Findings

The structure of the therapeutic programme, the residents' careers and their management and staff–resident boundaries were not considered to represent areas of noteworthy difference among the three TC-based services studied. The findings that follow therefore are those structural and cultural aspects that the organisational researchers considered most starkly demonstrated major convergences and divergences between the new units and Henderson, namely, staff profile, flattened hierarchy, and therapeutic engagement.

STAFF PROFILE

According to seniors interviewed at Webb House and its parent Trust, a match was intended between Henderson and Webb House's staff profile. However, during the period of the study there remained some differences, which require interpretation. There were relatively fewer nursing staff, and in particular fewer senior nursing staff, at Webb House. The Webb House pattern exhibited a flatter hierarchy, conforming to the principle of bringing management down to the lowest practical level. In terms of medical staffing, there was no Senior House Officer or Senior Registrar, and a full-time consultant post was only filled in April 2002 (18 months after opening). Senior staff did not wish to emulate the Henderson, as they felt it was over-medicalised for a socio-therapeutic setting. These variations appear to be legitimate modulations on the basic model, in keeping with the basic philosophy and responsive to local context.

The staff profile at Main House was similar to Henderson's, although this was because the Henderson happened to add a Senior Nurse post in the later stages of the replication project, bringing it closer to the Main House profile. The hierarchical structure at Main House, however, was more defined with additional tiers of middle management and a more specified line management system. From their interviews with staff, the researchers reported that the leadership did not wish to replicate what they perceived as an unclear organisational structure at the Henderson.

FLATTENED HIERARCHY

Webb House displayed some mismatches with the day-to-day management practices of the Henderson, especially in the first nine months of operation. Many of their staff had worked in vertically managed mainstream mental health organisations. A key issue therefore was how to ensure such individual professional accountability, but in a more collectively run organisation. Senior staff paradoxically tried to 'authorise' junior team members to claim authority to enact a flattened hierarchy. Moves towards democratisation were only slowly accomplished.

Hierarchical boundaries at Webb House were apparent, with staff allocated to groups by the Director and Lead Nurse but with the expectation that this should become a process managed later on by the staff team as a whole. Despite numerous attempts by seniors to facilitate activity by team members, in practice, allocation still depended on the Lead Nurse. By Year 2, however, more junior staff were leading on non-routine matters, as well as on more routinised decision-making. The researchers' interpretation was that Webb House progressively shifted towards a 'flatter hierarchy', after the early set up phase.

Main House demonstrated more mismatches than Webb House from the Henderson model. One early departure was the creation of a forum separate from the staff team for clinical managers' supervision, thus extracting supervision of more senior members from the full team. During member checking, seniors represented this as an opportunity for them to digest material before contributing to team supervision. To other staff, however, the supervision forum was a way of reaching a management view prior to discussion with staff – the antithesis of Henderson practice. Unlike the other two sites, at the request of the management group, the member checking exercise at Main House included a prior meeting with them, followed by a second meeting with the full team, at which seniors were also present.

Also, at Main House, from the reported accounts of junior staff interviewed, there appeared to be only modest budgetary delegation by managers, for example in relation to clinical 'work group' activities. During member checking, senior staff claimed that there was a higher degree of financial delegation, yet this was contested by junior staff members. At Henderson, such delegation is part of therapy, as residents feel empowered by the ability to make such financial decisions. The autonomy of junior staff was undermined by their belief that proposals for expenditure needed to be ratified by seniors. This was unlike practices at Henderson (and to a lesser extent) Webb House, where more budgetary matters were devolved.

Decisions about deployment of staff in the programme of therapeutic activities at Main House departed from practice at the Henderson, where these matters are decided through discussion by the staff team. There was a mix of team and managerial decisions, which left many staff puzzled. At interview, some staff expressed powerlessness and disappointment that the more democratic mode of working in the Henderson model had not been enacted. While not authoritarian, the managerial style at Main House was less democratic than at the other two sites. Senior staff suggested this was because of the rigours of establishing a new organisation, given the need to ensure unit safety and proper risk management.

THERAPEUTIC ENGAGEMENT

In the early months at Webb House, there was more individualisation of problems, with problems seen as the properties of individuals rather than of community dynamics, than was the norm at Henderson. In several community meetings, the Director and the Lead Nurse tried to engage residents to consider the wider significance of individual difficult behaviour for the whole community. Yet the community continued to engage with individual residents, asking them to 'talk about their problem'.

By Year 2, at Webb House, there was considerable progress towards Henderson's TC approach. Staff moved from being outside observers to being members of a community sharing opportunities for growth and development. The resident group took on a fuller, more proactive role, with a firmer sense of a collective responsibility for the running of the community and therapy. This was evident in day-to-day debates and decisions, actively taken up as 'learning materials'. Early crises or critical incidents enabled staff and residents to draw lessons and learn, congruent with the Henderson model. One example of organisational learning was when the Top Three/duty staff structure broke down one night in relation to the discharging of a resident from the TC. There was a loss of structure among Top Three and duty staff who were separately pursuing solutions, leading to an unhelpful escalation of events. The subsequent internal review concluded that the situation could have been better managed – with possibly different outcomes – had staff understood events in terms of the wider psychodynamic context of the community.

Residents at Webb House exhibited fewer learning behaviours at first, but this pattern slowly changed. By Year 2, residents were more vocal in community meetings, with less input from staff. This included a more sophisticated exploration of problems by residents: for example, more junior residents supporting more senior residents at times of heightened distress prior to their leaving, exploring risks of self-harm and future support options. Structures were being used in the service of enquiry rather than to apply punitive rules (as in the earlier days of the unit). By Year 2, key working practices (such as the daily staff handovers) had more resemblance to those at the Henderson. Talk often included the phrase 'could relate to', emphasising connections across the community. A wider range of staff was facilitating work with residents and engaging in more self-reflective talk. Overall, the community had a more mature and Henderson-like feel.

Main House rejected the role of senior residents known in the Henderson model as 'Top Three'. They still elected residents to work on behalf of the community with staff but these would instead be known as 'Resident Representatives' ('Res Reps'). This was part of establishing local ownership, explained in terms of rejecting Henderson's language with its militaristic roots and authoritarian connotations. This rejection appeared to be resident-led, their claiming that all were equal. In so doing, Main House rejected an important component of the model, wherein the flattened hierarchy on the staff side is counterbalanced by a definite hierarchy on the residents' side. As a result, the take-up of responsibility by senior residents at Main House was not robust. This problem of lack of responsibility was not owned by the resident group and was only picked up by a staff member. Unlike the Henderson, there was no listing of residents in chronological order of entry in any public manner (such as on a notice board in the community meeting room as at Henderson), so no very visible sense of seniority. During important meetings about elections, there was no differentiation regarding eligibility for residents' posts based on seniority or length of stay (residency) in the TC.

Over time, resident–resident interactions and challenges in Main House became more common. However, well into Year 2, residents regularly appeared to subvert therapy by engaging in power contests with staff. For example, there was a major contest about whether residents could change light bulbs in their bedrooms, or whether this was an offence against community and Trust rules in that light bulbs had to be replaced by Trust electricians, even if that meant waiting a week. At one point, 12 of the 18 residents came forward to admit light bulb changing offences, raising the spectre of a non-viable community if they were all discharged. There was some glee among the six other residents, who thought that they had their peers' fate in their hands. They were outvoted by staff, who voted to retain the residents. What is of interest, however, is not that this problem arose (power struggles are not unusual in any TC and can be used as opportunities for community learning) but how it was treated. Here, the matter was treated as a problem solved by invoking a rule and adopting a voting strategy to retain members. During member checking, it was reported that staff had later reflected on this incident. The so-called 'treatability' rule (allowing the community to assess and potentially discharge a resident thought not to be working authentically, yet not breaking rules that would threaten his or her continued membership of the TC) was little used in this period.

Such incidents suggested to the researchers that the 'culture of enquiry' at Main House was frail at this time. Though this developing TC held summit meetings, there was no standing procedure whereby items were fed into the community meeting and shared with the community. This suggested a lower priority was being given to the idea of the 'community as doctor' at Main House. Community and staff meetings were focused on the problems of individuals rather than community dynamics. As well as this tendency to individualise problems, staff were not using much of Henderson vocabulary that emphasised communalism within day-to-day practice.

Discussion

The easier dimension against which to evaluate replication is through structures and procedures rather than cultural aspects. Both new sites showed some differences from the Henderson in terms of staffing structures. At Webb House these could be seen as adaptations to local conditions or as principled departures designed to reach the same ends. Structures and procedures were largely 'Henderson-like'. At Main House, probably still more egalitarian than most mental health services, the authority structure was more hierarchical and the seniority structure among residents differed. Major decision-making was concentrated at the top, with middle management being treated as intermediaries for downward communication, and there was less consensus decision-making. This divergence was not limited to the set-up phase – Main House later moved towards a sharper hierarchy to ensure 'operational effectiveness', for example, concerning risk management). The standard (hierarchical) procedures of the host Trust reached deeply into work practices here.

The harder dimension of replication to evaluate related to the culture and values, as enacted in key working practices. Here again, Main House was relatively distinct, being more likely to define problems as properties of individuals to be remedied by the expert interventions of staff, hence (as noted above) the notion of 'community as doctor' was weak. A further difference was the weaker use of challenging behaviour, disagreements and dissensus as important therapeutic resources from which the community might learn and individuals develop psychologically. At Main House, such matters tended to be regarded more as being troublesome. To the organisational researchers, there was a relatively high congruence between patterns of working at the Henderson and Webb House but not so much between these and Main House. The researchers posited three possible explanations for this.

The first explanation lay in the distinctive and more experiential approach to replication adopted in Webb House. At Webb House, following their recruitment of Henderson staff (past and present), there was a strategy to export the model via identified 'culture carriers'. For example, three staff were recruited to key positions in the residential service (including the key post of Lead Nurse) and ex-Henderson residents – Volunteers – were recruited into development groups. This may have been a particularly potent approach to replication. These people were observed to be important members of the organisation during the first 18 months of services. Democratic TC philosophy requires organic, democratic 'replication', and a reliable method might be one that exports the model via people who serve to carry the culture. This is likely to be applicable for any model of care or organisation that is rooted in a specific expressed value-base and philosophy.

Second, Main House was the setting at which the procedures of the host NHS Trust reached most deeply into the service. These emphasised the development of codified systems of assessment, risk management and professional accountability, seen as normal in most mental health settings. They were embraced by senior staff there as ensuring effective management capacity. Such professional pressures, although also evident in the Henderson in the late 1990s, had been adapted there to be more consistent with the democratic TC model. At Henderson the TC model sat uneasily with this formalisation process, which bureaucratised decision-making and eroded tacit and collective systems of working.

Third, and critically, the underlying therapeutic ideology and pre-history at Main House was less receptive to Henderson ideas than at Webb House. Democratic TCs are value-laden organisations and there is no single agreed approach. Ideological differences between TC models were noted by the researchers to have been present throughout the project. According to them, these fed into inter-site power struggles and limited the effectiveness of replication strategies which did not take such ideological and political considerations into account.

Evidence from the clinical progress and health economic strands

The primary aim of the research was to evaluate whether replication of the Henderson Model at the two new sites had been successful. The specific objectives of the clinical progress strand were: to compare whether the three sites attracted and admitted similar patients; and to compare whether clinical changes in the three sites followed similar patterns. The specific objectives of the health economic strand were: to compare the cost of service provision at each of the three sites; and to compare whether changes in the resource use of patients before and after TC treatment followed similar patterns.

Research method

The study was a naturalistic, prospective cohort study (non-controlled). All consecutive referrals to each of the three sites and all consecutive admissions over a 12-month period from August 2001 were invited to participate. For the clinical progress strand data were collected for seven time points (referral, admission, and three-monthly intervals to 15 months post admission) to reflect patients' clinical status prior to treatment, during treatment and post discharge. The three primary collection points were referral, admission and 15 months post admission. The primary outcome measures were the Borderline Syndrome Index (BSI) (Conte et al. 1980) and length of stay in the TC.

For the health economic strand, data were collected at nine time points (admission and, for patients discharged from the democratic TC, at three-monthly intervals to a maximum of 24 months post admission) to reflect resource use in the year before and the year after treatment. A self-report service use questionnaire was developed for the purposes of this study, which collected resource use data on all service providing sectors (health care, social services and criminal justice). A costing exercise was conducted to identify, measure and value all resources used at each of the three democratic TCs to reflect resource use during treatment. This included preparation, selection, treatment and aftercare provided by both outreach and inpatient services. All costs were calculated for the financial year 2002/2003. Statistical analyses compared each of the two new sites with the original site (Henderson Hospital).

Results

Six hundred and fifty-nine patients, who had been consecutively referred to the three services, were approached by the researchers for participation in the study. Three hundred and forty-nine of these responded positively and consented to take part. One hundred and twenty-nine of this group were subsequently admitted to one of the TCs (out of a total of 164 admissions during the period of the study) and 97 completed the follow-up assessment at the 15-month point.

The three sites had similar patterns of referrals and admissions and there were no significant differences between the three sites in length of stay and clinical changes measured by BSI. The total costs per bed day were not significantly different across each of the sites. Overall there was a significant reduction in costs post-discharge in all three sites. The change in total costs per patient achieved at the two new sites was not significantly different from those achieved at the Henderson Hospital. A linear regression was conducted of changes in costs against changes in BSI, which showed that the greater the change in BSI score, the greater the cost reduction.

Discussion

The independent researchers considered that Strands 2 and 3, clinical progress and health economic, had achieved the aim of testing the replication of the two new democratic TCs based on the Henderson Hospital. According to them, their main results indicated that Henderson's model had been successfully replicated to the two new sites in terms of the primary outcome measures, length of stay and changes in Borderline Syndrome Index scores. The researchers acknowledged that the study was limited, in that follow-up was necessarily short (hence numbers of subjects in the sample relatively small due to the anticipated slow throughput of patients at the three sites). However, the research design allowed the findings from the two strands to be integrated. The researchers considered that the positive and significant association between reduced costs and clinical progress offered cross-strand validation. These findings, taken together, allowed the researchers to form conclusions that they saw as robust. The researchers further concluded that sufficient replication had occurred to allow the three TC-based services to be used as a single treatment arm in any future outcome study.

Conclusions

The whole research project was set up to assess whether or not replication had been achieved. Its three-stranded methodology reflected the complexity of the subject matter. Therefore in addition to a qualitative organisational strand (evaluated by an ethnographic method), there were two quantitative stands – clinical progress and health economic. It would be in taking the results of these three together that ultimate sense might be made and a conclusive answer to the replication question provided.

The quantitative strands' researchers concluded that their results had formed a relatively stringent test of the replication – one that the replication project appeared to 'pass'. However, the results of the qualitative research, deriving as it does from a different paradigm, could not yield a categorical 'pass–fail' answer. There was no agreed method of pooling the results from all three strands. The second and third strands, whose methodology was shared and whose sampling was thus contemporaneous, could complement one another. Integrating these results with those of the organisational strand, however, was not straightforward, not least since there was only little overlap in the timing of data collection between the first and the latter two strands. The potential advantage of this multi-stranded approach, therefore, was not fully realised since the project took longer than envisaged to deliver and there was insufficient funding, hence time, to achieve all of the original ambitions of the project.

More funding and time would have been required to explore ways of integrating the results of the three stands. It therefore remains an individual matter as to how much to value the findings from any of the three strands on their own and how far to attempt to amalgamate supporting or contradictory material from another stand in respect of the question of replication. The reader will therefore need to decide for himself or herself what is their verdict, taking into account also the subjective 'findings' reported by the author in this book and the appended views of two service users. The latter's comments were unsolicited and are provided as 'the last word' in this chapter:

> We are not all people who are ashamed to say we have been in these units…the experience I have had, and blatantly the one making the highest degree of difference to my life and relationships, was the year I spent in Webb House…I can see the value, my friends can see the value and I am constantly using what I learned and gained there to continue to grow in this way.

> Pre-Main House I'd written myself off, as had many others, but now I have a life which is full of progress. I'm just coming out of a deep and protracted depression (6 months) but did not revert to psychotropic meds and managed (just) to keep my PD behaviours in check (only just, but I did). If all of you other TCs out there can help one or two others to come as far as I have, you all deserve a momentary head swell to feel proud of what you have achieved.

CHAPTER SEVEN

A Last Supper

Introduction

It is not entirely clear what marked the end of our replication feast. At the time of starting to write this chapter – October 2004 – the final reports of the independent researchers (clinical progress and health economic strands) are still subject to the peer review process – two broadly positive and one decidedly negative view having been received (and responded to by the relevant researchers). In this sense, perhaps the festivities are still not over. In another sense, however, the meal table is already being cleared, even if there are still some of us sitting around it! NSCAG had decided (in October 2003) that the funding of the national service for severe personality disorders should stop in April 2005 (later revised to 2006: see below). Beyond this point, responsibilities for funding would pass to local commissioners – Primary Care Trusts – some 300 or so in total for England. The latter would decide whether or not to continue to purchase. This state of affairs thus resembles the 'marketplace' situation, which Henderson had been keen to escape prior to submitting its bid to NSCAG.

The Department of Health's current policy emphasises the inclusion of personality disordered individuals. The latter are (at last) deemed to be equally deserving of mental healthcare as are other patients – 'Personality disorder: No longer a diagnosis of exclusion' (NIMHE 2003). Their guidance document also mentions Henderson, Main and Webb, though does not specify the role of such tertiary services. Implicitly, it endorses their inclusion as part of a comprehensive range of services for personality disorder (see Norton, Healy and Lousada 2005). So, at a time when the DH acknowledges the need for more services for personality disorder, it is ironic that the future of Birmingham and Henderson's democratic therapeutic community-centred services are in jeopardy and the residential therapeutic community in Crewe – Webb House – has already been forced to close (14 July 2004). This chapter thus attempts to identify how this state of affairs might be understood.

Mulling it over

The original deal was for Henderson to undertake what was referred to at the time as 'replication', although this term does not do justice to the complex set of dynamic as well as static factors involved. In order that replication could be fairly judged to have been achieved, or not, there had to be an external, independent evaluation. The research design included a descriptive, organisational limb and two others – clinical progress (a phrase chosen to distinguish the research question from that of 'effectiveness' or 'outcome') and health economic (essentially a detailed evaluation of service costs and cost-offset). In 1997, the commissioners, NSCAG, had apparently been sufficiently satisfied by the evidence base of Henderson Hospital to allocate funding (over the years since April 1998, totalling approximately £30 million) for the pump-priming of these new PD developments, an undertaking not before made by this national funding body and not without its critics (see Kisely 1999). This new research, however, would not directly add to the sum of knowledge about TC treatment outcome per se, since its aim was a more modest one – merely to detect replication. Limited though they might be, its findings would, so we had been led to believe, bear on the question of future national funding for the three services – in fact, the door had been left open by NSCAG for them to fund the development of further similar services, so as to fulfil the original brief of 'Hendersons' in the North, South, East and West.

Well, at times, the original deal was barely discernible. There had been precious little recognition by commissioners that setting up, at a distance, two specialist services for such difficult-to-manage and at times dangerous clients was problematic and requiring of support and sensitivity. So it had not been helpful, for example, that the costs of the three services were continually compared, questioned and challenged while the health economic 'experiment' (set up to evaluate this aspect among others – see Chapter 6) was still running. Part of the original Government interest in the project had stemmed from the fact that there was ignorance about the relative costs of setting up and running ostensibly the same service but in different parts of the country. There was genuine interest therefore (or so we had been told) in understanding any identifiable differences.

There seemed to be no awareness, however, since NSCAG were attempting to manipulate costs to be the same in each of the three different localities, that such interference could potentially jeopardise the very research that they themselves had instigated. Their repeated requests for more and more detailed breakdown of performance activity and costings also simply took valuable human resources away from the authentic management tasks of these young services – and there were many such tasks. This number-crunching, much of it seemingly for its own sake, seldom appeared to yield any tangible outputs, let alone benefits. It was also clear from meetings with them, that some of the data were only cursorily inspected by the commissioners, if at all.

Little or no credence was given to the difficulty of the developmental work in terms of the work-related anxiety carried by staff working in the three services, especially in the two new developments. (It should not be forgotten that Henderson itself had been – half of the time – without its Director and some of its senior staff, i.e. those involved in the HDT.) Worse than this, from Henderson's perspective, was to follow. Through NSCAG's account of recent history, it was as if the Reed Report had quite erroneously identified Henderson's service as being of value and relevance to the needs of 'Difficult and Offender Patients' (Reed 1994). NSCAG commissioners suggested, without comparative data, that our PD patients were less severe than those treated in day hospitals and our treatment no more successful, implying that there might have been no justification for commissioning a residential service as this specialised service for severe PD. Perhaps, in their (indirectly stated) view, Reed had been wrong to recommend more Hendersons.

Even the tragic event of a homicide perpetrated by one ex-resident of one of the new services on another – albeit some months after each had (separately) left that facility – did not appear to challenge the commissioners' view that we treated only good prognosis cases. Then, it was as if they hit upon it – our risk-assessment processes must be suspect! Therefore, in October 2003, given barely ten days' notice and precious little explanation, the Chief Executives of the three services were informed that an independent expert had been appointed to inspect the three elements of the national service. This was to evaluate how well (or badly) risk was assessed and managed.

In the circumstances, such a course of action was not unreasonable, although the length of time that had elapsed between the untoward event and the discharge from treatment was arguably great. Therefore many factors, quite independent of the TC service itself, would have been operative and potentially influential in the interim period. Ironically, the first of these three evaluations was of Henderson. To be fair, there could be logic in seeing how the prototype service dealt with matters of risk before visiting the derivative services. Perhaps what was in question was something intrinsic to the democratic TC model, which might lie behind the tragic event – if that were their motive. It would have helped to have understood more of the reasoning behind this sudden inspection – for there to have been greater transparency.

Our collective sense within the national severe PD service, call it paranoia, was that NSCAG hoped that fault would be found in us in order to justify closure. The whole replication project would all have been a ghastly mistake but, with the TC beast lying slain, everybody could now rest easy at night. Too poetic and hyperbolic, no doubt. At any rate, an early closure of the Units could mean that later difficult decisions (the need to evaluate the scientifically derived data from the independent research) might be avoided. Indeed, the wait for the research findings would no longer have to be endured. In fact, we had received requests from NSCAG to provide them with 'headline' findings, ahead of the agreed timing of the research. They seemed to have developed a convenient amnesia about the date when the study would report – not a state secret. So there we were, in October 2003, with inspections under way into clinical governance arrangements, especially risk assessment and management processes and procedures. We were to find out what they would reveal, though not straightaway.

We had been told that the report's findings, which would be delivered to NSCAG in early December, would be made available to us. On the face of it, it must be said that such a plan was sensible, given the possibility – if not likelihood – that if something untoward were discovered, it might require urgent attention. It was therefore odd, once the external report had been submitted, that it took more than three months for this document to be processed 'centrally' before it was finally released to the Chief Executives of the three Trusts. It only arrived then after repeated attempts by the Trusts to find out from NSCAG what delays might have been encountered and what adverse findings there might have been. In relation to Henderson, four concerns were identified:

- the need to do more to prevent early dropout from treatment
- the need to revisit the issue of 'ligature points', i.e. easy sites from which to enact self-strangulation
- the need to comply with separate-sex bathroom accommodation
- the need to do more to understand, and if possible alleviate, inequalities of access to the service by patients from ethnic minorities.

These four aspects, important as they are, were offset by the praise heaped upon the three services, and indirectly, on the democratic TC model. However, given the importance and urgency of attending to at least one of the above matters (namely, that related to ligature points), it remains difficult to comprehend the mentality that withholds the findings of such an inquiry. To us, the delay seemed to contradict the sense of urgency that there had been to get the inspection carried out. Perhaps NSCAG had to 'tick some box'. Perhaps this had been their paramount concern (i.e. initiating the inspection, regardless of its subsequent contents), and we had been wrong to attribute to NSCAG the motive of wanting to close the services.

In essence, the inspector found Henderson to be providing a safe and therapeutic environment with clear rules and boundaries. Further than this he indicated that Henderson's TC approach had much to teach the mainstream mental health world on how to manage disturbance. Henderson's relationship with its host Trust was also acknowledged to be good with a well-integrated programme of clinical governance-related activities. In common with Main and Webb House, which were also inspected, the units were reported as having unparalleled experience and expertise in helping people with personality disorder and, together, as playing a vital role as part of a comprehensive approach to personality disorder services. Helpfully to us, the inspector's report also included what it referred to as 'key challenges over the next year' that faced the three national services. These concerned the need for a smooth transfer of funding from NSCAG, recognising there was a requirement for detailed joint planning and a service development strategy in order to effect this transfer.

Returning to October 2003, alongside the timetable for 'external' inspection there was launched a timetable for transferring the funding of the national service from NSCAG to Primary Care Trusts (PCTs), as if the existence of an inspection itself sounded the death knell, irrespective of its subsequent, generally positive, findings. The three NSCAG-appointed local 'lead' commissioners tasked with overseeing the process, which allowed a period of 16 months to re-commission, acknowledged that the time was too short. It was not clear, to those of us now sidelined, by being excluded from face-to-face meetings with NSCAG, just what or who was attempting to drive this process at such a reckless rate. The findings of both the research and 'risk' inspection were yet to be reported. From the autumn, the DH had begun a programme of restructuring, shedding (by one way or another) up to a third of its staff. Perhaps it was this that provided the impetus for such thoughtless action.

Alternatively, NIMHE's agenda might have been well served by a cash injection of funds, which could result from any redistribution of the costs represented by our national PD service. The implementation of the NIMHE's guidance on PD services and related training, *Personality Disorder: No Longer a Diagnosis of Exclusion* (2003), could not enjoy protected funding through the PCT route. 'Guidance' meant simply that and there was no requirement that local commissioners would spend the 'new PD money' on PD patients, or even on those with severe mental illness. Therefore, PCTs might benefit from any redistribution of funds currently tied up (in what we were repeatedly told was our luxurious and expensive national service). They could use this to match NIMHE's new money, which would result in more local ring-fenced PD money at least in the short term – a deal that could have been attractive to them.

The short time-scale for transfer of commissioning, and its method of implementation, did spell out the end of the national service for severe PD, as a single entity. The timing was cynical, ironic, being only months after the launch of the NIMHE guidance document, in which it was acknowledged that TCs had a part to play. Indeed, three such were acknowledged to be sites of 'notable practice'. How could it be, with so few months having elapsed following publication, that three PD services – only a matter of five years after having been described by the DH as 'centres of excellence' – would now be floated on a local commissioning system that would be unable to cope with them? Why the indecent haste? Was this a conspiracy or cock-up?

Room 101

Even ahead of what was acknowledged by most involved to be too short a time to communicate effectively with the 300 or so PCTs, one of the hosting Trusts decided to close their residential TC. Instead it was to re-deploy the staff resource to support 'local developments'– the thrust of NIMHE's guidance in relation to secondary level care for PD. The central thinking appeared to be that existing specialist PD services could be safely demolished before the new ones had been built. We wondered how you safely demolish a therapeutic setting for difficult and offender patients, without incurring unreasonable levels of risk and without making suitable re-provision. Whether such a question was ever asked or answered centrally we do not know.

Come the appointed time for the plans for transfer of commissioning to be presented to NSCAG (March 2004), no objection appears to have been raised to the proposed closure of one inpatient resource – Webb House. This would have more than just a local effect on PD service provision, already acknowledged by NIMHE to be very patchy or non-existent in many parts of the country. Things were moving fast, albeit in a largely destructive manner. Clearly, managers and commissioners can demolish services faster than clinicians can create them – if this contention were ever in doubt.

The upsetting effect on those of us who had worked so hard (and I would add so effectively and, arguably, so efficiently) to set up the new PD services cannot be overstated. It is noteworthy that, at a meeting (January 2004) among the three services to review plans, in the light of the forthcoming transfer of funding to PCTs, it had taken over an hour for the fact of the decision to close Webb House to be communicated by their senior staff to the rest of us present – their opposite numbers. Remember, many of us had, by this time, worked closely together for a period of over six years. Yet such was the personal impact of this impending communication about closure that it could not easily be spoken. And, of course, once spoken, the rest of us could not readily take it in.

The sense of disbelief, almost unreality for me, was only heightened when it turned out that my hotel room that night, where we were staying outside Warwick, was Room 101 – auspicious or what? Numbness, sadness and outrage, by degrees and in turn, got expressed that evening. We did not know where best to focus our individual and collective energies. Should we try to overturn what had been decided about Webb House? How much should we attempt to band together, in the belief that we might be still a stronger unit – as one rather than three? It was difficult to summon the energy even to eat supper. Yet it also seemed important that we should not see ourselves as total failures, though our 'all-for-one-and-one-for-all' days seemed a distant memory. I felt that, at least, our gathering in Warwick should recognise and not deny the success we had achieved, in having set out to do what, at least originally, the Government had also desired of us. Although we were keen to know what the independent research would reveal, our clinical impressions of the services were that they could make a beneficial difference, at least to some of our residents' lives. We did not know, of course, if such views would be validated by the research.

In an attempt to lift spirits, my own as much as (or even more than) those of others, I ordered champagne – not the best but not just sparkling wine either. This was without doubt one of the better decisions that I made during the course of this project. We toasted ourselves, not least since there was precious little likelihood that anybody else would! I think it helped a bit, at the time. That evening one of the assembled group fainted – not from excess bubbly. The incident appeared to be related critically to what was being done to our PD service. It had felt a bit like a 'last supper' for this team that had created the national PD service.

Early the following morning, a small number of us had a pre-breakfast meeting (and one had already been on the hotel's treadmill by then, as if that of the NHS were insufficiently demanding). Unsurprisingly, the negative moods had persisted but there was agreement about engaging with the questions posed the evening before. One of our number accepted the nomination to chair a brainstorming session, during which we attempted to pool our thoughts. (We numbered 12 – three Business Managers, three Lead Nurses, three other senior staff and the three Directors.) This would help us to decide whether we were 'one', 'three' or 'three in one' and if we should accept the closure of Webb House as a *fait accompli*. We would try to agree what might be done collectively and separately. These deliberations took place with reasonably good grace, for the most part, and with more enthusiasm than we might have been entitled to expect from one another, under the circumstances.

Back in Sutton, after this dispiriting Warwick meeting, the main task was to keep concentrating on the clinical needs within Henderson. We needed to sustain our service, while feeling unappreciated and unvalued by the wider 'system', the effects of the intoxicating bubbles now having long since worn off. At Henderson, we continued to experience staff shortages, which had meant the rota staff undertaking much more night shift-work than was usual or desirable, in terms of offering clinical continuity and job satisfaction. In the residential service, we had a locum Clinical Lead in post (John Stevens), following the departure of the previous incumbent (Alex Esterhuyzen) at the end of October 2003. This post was not filled full-time, necessitating me to withdraw from my academic sessions to make up the shortfall.

In passing, it should be noted that the Henderson team worked together extremely effectively during this period of acute staffing shortage. There was much more blurring of roles and flattening of the hierarchy than was customary even at the Henderson. It was fortunate that quite a number of the staff were relatively new, hence not significantly invested in the wider national PD service. (The plan to induct all staff into the three services, to indicate involvement in a 'supra-system', although thought to be appropriate, had never really caught on.) Fortunately, therefore, the attention of these newer staff was focused on the clinical work, though there was also disquiet amongst them as to their longer-term job security, given the commissioning uncertainty.

Back in the routine of clinical work, some of us were periodically feeling torn between helping out the supra-system of the national service and keeping our own system afloat. At Henderson, we were exercised and taxed by these twin demands. Yet, the demands of the clinical work dictated that we attend more to our own situation, a state of affairs which seemed to be mirrored in the other two services. However cathartic the Warwick meeting brainstorming had been (and however painful), once back 'home' that is where charity began. Worryingly, it took some effort to remember what had been decided as a result of the brain-storming and to position this in the overall list of Henderson priorities.

The list, at Henderson, was topped by the need to work together with our designated local mental health lead commissioner to try to ensure our own future to the extent that this might be possible. This was really the only game in town. Yet, it became clear that, with a little thought, it might also be possible to campaign on both fronts. It was also possible, as we had identified at the brain-storming, to make representations to a range of bodies that might be more or less influential (for example, the Royal College of Psychiatrists) and from a number of different positions (for example, political) and roles (citizen, professional).

From my position, as citizen, I could write to my MP, particularly to complain about the closure of Webb House. I could comment upon what might be seen as a waste of tax-payers' money – my money – as well as a threat to na-tionally needed services. As Henderson's future was also in the balance, I could mention its potential loss, which could impact negatively locally. I could also comment on the potential loss of specialist skills, at a time when the Government were identifying the need for more such. And I could legitimately copy this letter to others. Those who had been involved in the research from the outset would recognise that this costly-to-set-up service was being potentially devastated with decommissioning decisions being taken ahead of the reporting of the research findings that had taken years to accumulate (and would be available in just a matter of months). The President of the Royal College of Psychiatrists would surely wish to be apprised of the situation, not least since he had links with NSCAG, although only relatively recently so. I felt moved to wonder if it had been 'stigma' towards an already stigmatised client group that could lie behind what otherwise appeared to be an unaccountable oversight – the closure of Webb House. Therefore, the Royal College lead of its anti-stigma campaign could be copied in. Fortuitously, the Mental Health Tsar had written on this very topic of stigma (in relation to PD) some years earlier, so he might wish to ponder this theory to account for the closure. My letter thus would have a wide circulation.

But I was also a doctor. I had colleagues who valued the work of Henderson and would say as much when alerted to the situation. I could also write, as doctor, to the All Party Mental Health Group, via its secretary who happened to be both Lord and psychotherapist. The primary aim was not to politicise the situation, at least not in a party political sense. This letter also served to be copied to other parties. I hoped that one result might be the formation of a loose network of interested parties. I approached past and present colleagues for advice, to ask how best to manage such a threatening situation. Many views on tactics were expressed, including those tactics described here. Voluntary bodies were approached. Serendipitously, via the Association of Therapeutic Communities there was an invitation to speak to the All Party group just referred to, though apparently not in relation to the letter sent to the House of Lords.

We still had not as yet used what we saw as a potential winning card – the residents or, at least, ex-residents! The ex-residents whose contact details we had from their days in the HDT were contacted to tell them the gloomy news. The reason for this was twofold. We wanted to enlist what support they might be willing and able to offer and we did not want them to hear of the potential closure via the grapevine, since this we thought would have been more upsetting. We had also informed the current Henderson residents, since some of these had been due to meet with those from other TCs and there was the possibility that they too would have heard it first from this source rather than from ourselves. From such a route (possibly implying our withholding such negative tidings) it would have been a short journey to residents believing that Henderson was sure to suffer a similar fate to that of Webb House. Therefore there was a need to inform them of the facts and to indicate something of the potential impact on our own service – from which, we believe, they were deriving therapeutic benefit.

Our Trust was clearly behind us, offering to set up a 'Commissioning Group' headed by the Director of Planning. This would coordinate the activities going on within Henderson and the wider Trust so that we could avoid duplication of effort and keep all parties in the picture with up-to-date information – at least that was the theory. This group related to the Henderson Project Group chaired by the mental health lead commissioner for London who had been tasked by NSCAG to identify future funding for Henderson. In turn, that group set up a 'Reference Group' comprising PCTs (i.e. local commissioners of whom there were over 120 who were relevant in the whole of the South East region), clinicians (some who had been referrers and some who had not referred, at least not recently), representatives of other tertiary PD services and service users ('experts by experience' – though not through Henderson's own service).

Supporting the whole commission-seeking enterprise were a firm of Health Service Consultants working (initially) under the direction of the mental health lead commissioner for London. It was the former's role to ensure that all the necessary paperwork was available; they drafted reports for meetings and in some instances presented the data and the arguments so that the potential new commissioners could understand that which they might be about to fund. The money that was at stake was £20,000 per PCT. Interestingly, one of the local PCT's commissioners considered this amount of money to be insufficient a sum, even to call a PCT board meeting. Yet the re-commissioning task had launched what seemed a huge flotilla of meetings, whose membership represented thousands of pounds of taxpayers' money each time we met. £20,000 was also an insufficient amount to set up any local service; it might have bought the better part of a Community Psychiatric Nurse or half of a junior doctor for a year. Pooled together of course it represented a whole tertiary level service – our service. The absence of just a few such £20,000 would seriously undermine the Henderson or Main House services.

Now what is going on?

For reasons that still remain obscure to me, the decision by NSCAG to hand over commissioning to PCTs in April 2005 was revoked (March 2004). The date for handover to the PCTs, a more realistic one, became April 2006. The President of the Royal College of Psychiatrists – part of the NSCAG board by virtue of his position – claimed to have argued successfully for the need for 'Hendersons' as part of the comprehensive range of PD services. Why the weight of this argument had not been felt earlier is not known, nor whether this argument had indeed been put earlier. The letter outlining the news to the three Chief Executives suggested that the reason related to the need for independent research findings, the expected date of arrival of which had been somehow forgotten.

The letter suggested that information about the reporting dates of the research was not available or perhaps not obtainable. Yet it would not have taken much to establish such knowledge. A telephone call to me or indeed to anybody involved in the research would have revealed the answer to the implied mystery. It was also implied that a failure to solve this simple mystery had led to a decision to decommission early. In fact, it was hard to understand what the mixture of tenses really meant. It might be thought that the words of such an important letter would have been chosen with care and with a view to imparting a clear message. In fact it was hard to know what the mixture of tenses could really mean. It concealed more than it conveyed. It might therefore have been intended to represent a convenient fig-leaf, behind which to hide the shameful fact that the time-scale for decommissioning was ill-judged.

So that was the 'good news'. We now had more time in which to find a solution to the commissioning conundrum. Why a conundrum? How complicated can commissioning arrangements be? Does it really take so many people, in so many meetings, to identify what in the end must be a simple mechanism? In fact, there is a limited range of possibilities. At one end is some form of 'top-slicing' for an agreed area, such as London (via 'specialist commissioning groups' agreeing with mental health leads). At the other is a 'cost per case' option. In between, there are varying mixtures of consortium groups (agreeing to co-commission for a given area) with 'cost per case' purchasing. To me, that captures the complexity. However, there seemed to be no will from the top to make some new purchasing arrangement happen. This to me was, and still is, surprising. The DH acknowledges that services for the PD client group are poor and that specialist PD services have a place in the range of treatments required – as argued both by the President to NSCAG (see above) and the NIMHE guidance document *Personality Disorder: No Longer a Diagnosis of Exclusion*.

Specialist commissioners then made it clear to the lead commissioners for London charged with finding Henderson's funding for the future (according to the latter's account) that they were not interested in hearing special pleading on behalf of an individual institution such as Henderson. They needed to know about its place and role in the provision of services to the relevant client group – not an unreasonable request. What was therefore required was the creation of a network of specialist services, in which it would need to be agreed that Henderson had a place – an entire (pan-London) service. This, rather than a single service entity, could attract specialist commissioning. This represented a much greater task to be undertaken by us but within the longer time frame. So, although there was now more time to identify funding, there was a bigger job to be done in identifying a severe PD service for London and the South East.

Worse was to follow, which in so many ways typified what was so difficult about this whole project to set up new services – 'events, dear boy, events', as Harold Macmillan had famously commented. 'Exit' events to be precise. When the good news of extended funding was announced, I had written to all concerned about not getting complacent and losing momentum. At that time, everybody seemed to agree that this was the right approach. But then, all eyes were taken off just about any ball that was moving in the relevant field! The lead mental health commissioner, to whom the bulk of the work had been delegated, was promoted and exited to the North of England. That person's boss had more pressing engagements to attend, so was not present to chair meetings that she had set up.

One of these was a key meeting of the Henderson Project Group with the Reference Group it had set up (it just had to be 1 April 2004). Apologies from the absent chair were only received at the last moment, meaning that those standing in had little warning and less time during which to prepare and replace, although, in the event, the meetings passed off tolerably well – albeit with only a tiny fraction of the total number of PCTs in attendance. Our Chief Executive failed to attend a three-monthly meeting with NSCAG (and the effective lead of the NIMHE PD programme) and also failed to send a deputy. 'I did not go' ran the email reply to my discreet enquiry for feedback from this meeting. (This was from someone who had given up time to attend an evening meeting with the All Party Mental Health Group not long before.) Our local man in the Trust on the day of our next monthly Commissioning Group meeting, which he was due to chair, sent apologies to this meeting, because 'something urgent had turned up'. What was now abundantly clear was that we were not urgent. Much of our local support had exited, temporarily, or at least become invisible.

Much of the NHS seems to be delivered with this paucity of control over management resources. As a result, there is a constant sense of 'fire-fighting' and only top priorities get real attention and only then for the barest minimum of time. Forward planning, and in particular support for new projects that require dedicated time and nurturing, do not really stand much chance of success. Once more we were dogged by a lack of commitment from higher 'management', not because they did not want to be supportive but because they were defeated by the system or allowed themselves to be so by not taking a more long-term perspective, getting better resourced or delegating more. I favour the first option.

In intensive care

The situation was getting complicated with the proliferation of meetings perhaps analogous to the sick patient admitted to an intensive care unit, with the 'life-lines' that often get established having the potential to distract from the actual patient. It becomes hard to discern the person because of the technology and instrumentation. (We had the Henderson Project Group, its Reference Group, the Trust's Commissioning Meeting, as well as Henderson's External Relations Group and Marketing Meeting – to name but the most relevant.) Henderson's clinical workload was hard to focus on with all the meetings with commissioners and related meetings. In an attempt to simplify matters, therefore, we merged our longstanding Henderson Marketing Meeting with the hastily constituted External Relations Group (ERG), set up to deal with the commissioning issues, to form the Marketing and External Relations Group (MERG). It was not very imaginative but kind of memorable. This new group's brief was in part to plan marketing strategy in relation to obtaining necessary external contacts and support in the event of further closure threats and in part to keep the wider staff team aware of and involved in the issues related to re-commissioning.

Our Director of Planning had been leading the monthly Commissioning Meeting, also attended by our Directorate medical lead and Service Manager, in addition to myself. This meeting, coordinating our Trust's response to feedback from the Henderson Project Group (higher up) and now from MERG (below), seemed to be useful in defining a consistent line and view from the Trust's perspective. However, it was difficult to keep abreast of the many other meetings that were instituted within the London commissioning scene and beyond. So many of the relevant 'structures' seemed to be emergent, rather than fixed, and not even all commissioners agreed about the function of the constituent parts! For example, the commissioners tasked with identifying the new commissioning arrangements appeared to disagree with the view of the external consultant they had hired about the role, hence relevance, of the Strategic Health Authorities, in relation to commissioning. The latter contended he had it as part of his brief – in a supervisory capacity – while the former contested this view. (Witnessing this type of situation made matters confusing to a humble clinician.) NSCAG and NIHME, if these could be distinguished at this time, seemed to be holding impromptu meetings with the 'lead' commissioner and somehow the plan to design a pan-London 'clinical network'(previously deemed necessary by London's commissioning powers-that-be) had been dropped. Confusingly, we heard that there would be too little time to develop this, even with the extension to 2006.

What, we asked, had happened to the requirement that Henderson's service would need to be seen within a network of tertiary services if it were to attract pan-London commissioning support? Well, we did not get an answer to this obvious and direct question. It was as if we just had to trust that 'they' knew what they were doing – 'Trust me, I'm a commissioner.' With such a lack of transparency and conflicting views, it was hard to feel trusting. But we had no other realistic options. It is true that we had had meetings with local MPs (two Liberal Democrats and one Conservative), all of whom had appeared interested and helpful – the election was not so very far off. They were keen to get debates in the House or questions tabled. We had also written to a 'Lord', who had tabled his own questions in the House, especially regarding the closure of Webb House. He had received the usual assurances, in language that hid at least half of the truth. For example, the 'new day services' referred to that the Webb staff would engage with have still not started to operate at the time of writing this. The tenor of the letter, though not the precise content, since there was little enough of this, appeared to be along the following lines. You can purchase many day services for the price of one residential unit – not contestable in financial terms. Necessarily, day services are better value for money than residential services – contestable.

We had not wanted to pursue this political route, however, unless forced to do so by the failure of the NHS processes described above, even though the meetings that took place failed to inspire confidence in commissioners because of their changing membership and the moving goalposts. Perhaps the commissioning task was more manageable, however, with our not having to invent a clinical network – though, independently, we had already started work on this with colleagues from the Cassel and Tavistock/Portman Clinics (see Norton *et al.* 2005).

Meetings followed meetings, and it started to become difficult to feed back to Henderson staff team so little progress from so much apparent external activity. In the meantime, following untoward events in the Trust, the financial position of South West London and St George's Mental Health NHS Trust deteriorated to an unprecedented extent – it never before had failed to 'balance its books'. This had two main effects on our position. The Director of Planning was removed from our Commissioning Meeting and associated meetings, so that he could concentrate on his main duties, i.e. to the wider Trust (August 2004) – not an unreasonable step for the Chief Executive to have taken. However, it meant that the Trust was no longer prepared to accept the previous level of financial risk posed by Henderson. Whereas many other specialist services had survived on a mix of 'consortium' and 'cost per case' funding, our Trust would no longer countenance this, so we were told informally.

We had previously been put in touch with an institution in the private sector – in fact a not-for-profit organisation, which was decidedly interested in taking us over. They viewed us as real value for money, actually quite cheap – 'We could add 15 per cent to those charges straight away.' They would use our 'badge', our 'good name' as they saw it, and would be willing to preserve, to an extent, much of our existing clinical practice and the terms and conditions of working for many of the staff. My reading of this, however, was that what was distinctive (and arguably thera-peutic) in our democratic TC approach would be quickly eroded or at least difficult to preserve. Almost certainly, so I imagined, we would be forced to take PD patients on psychotropic medication, on sections of the Mental Health Act (i.e. those compelled to receive treatment), and who knew what else? Our beds would be kept full, at all costs, and we would be treating a different clientele for which we were not prepared and for which we had no experience and no evidence base. It would not only be likely that we would have ceased to be 'Henderson', as we knew ourselves, but that we would be undertaking riskier business – overall, a very high-risk strategy to pursue, in more ways than one.

By June 2004, it was abundantly clear to me, from my attendance at the seemingly unending series of meetings with commissioners (including the periodic meetings with NSCAG, who now wished to meet twice as often to review progress against our 'service level agreement' contract) that there was not a 'no change' option for Henderson. This was not necessarily a bad thing in itself. Webb House we knew was due to close shortly (July 2004). Main House, we had heard, was in the process of offering a menu of services from which their local commissioners might choose. (N.B. Communication among the three limbs of our once proud national service was almost non-existent, as if the limbs were already severed.)

In our Trust (and with only a narrow circulation), we had viewed the private/charity sector takeover of Henderson option seriously, but as a 'Plan B'. However, after a discussion limited to a small number of senior staff, it seemed that this was not a tenable option in that it would have little or no support from those who wished to do more than simply preserve the Henderson 'logo'. We thus needed to develop other fallback positions. We looked therefore more closely at what Main House were proposing – downsizing, opening a day service, taking patients on psychotropic medication, etc., etc. We did not see this as either attrac-tive or necessarily within our compass to provide safely, given our existing expertise and track record – possibly a too modest or conservative self-assess-ment. Elderly Henderson was perhaps too set in its ways, and attractive options for us would need to be both clearly feasible and at least partially desirable to our current staff – the product of democratisation in action, at least to a limited extent. Plan B thus was relegated to Plan C and further detailed thinking about alternative Plan Bs was progressed.

We considered some fairly drastic options in spite of our old age and conser-vatism. One such, deriving from what Webb House had found itself undertaking in its terminal phase, was to become a service for the detailed (six weeks) assessment of complex PD cases, those who they would have previously tried to engage and treat within a residential but not primarily a 'treatment' setting. We also considered adopting the Cassel strategy of shorter (six months) residential stay and longer outpatient aftercare, though this flew in the face of our research findings that there was increasing benefit shown up to nine months – this would therefore need to be the level to which any treatment were abbreviated. We wondered if we should by-pass the residents, thereby relatively distempering them at least in the short term, and allow staff alone to decide who should be admitted. After a probationary period, residents would then vote to decide if the probationer residents should stay – a kind of deferred selection process. None of these ideas or proposals gained much support. However, they were retained as Plan Bs. In being under our control, these were more attractive than Plan C, the takeover option.

Meanwhile, we were concentrating on making Plan A as competitive as possible. This represented the least change option, although it would encompass significant changes, both in terms of Henderson's internal organisation – especially involving a much closer working relationship between those delivering the Outreach function and the residential staff – and with the wider system, i.e. other tertiary-level specialist PD services and also other agencies related to the PD clientele. The idea was that we would attempt to create a 'managed clinical network' (Norton *et al.* 2005). This network of tertiary services would plug into the secondary-level psychiatric services, including the specialist PD services which were being funded by NIMHE-related money. Some of the changes suggested by the external inquiry into our risk assessment and management processes would also be incorporated. So by the height of summer 2004 we were accepting in the wider staff team that change was inevitable and that we would be putting maximal effort into maintaining the residential service but making it better fit for purpose within the changing PD and wider secondary-tier mental health services landscape. (In this venture we were being helped by two co-opted ex-residents.) The hope was that our eventual package of changes would be attractive to commissioners to fund.

For a long time NSCAG had been extremely keen for us to change. This attitude was difficult to comprehend now, however, since they wanted, and were, to be rid of us. They seemed determined to support us to get new commissioners, but at the same time were broadcasting a message that, as we were, we were not purchasable! They did not accept that this was a valid construction of their position, or indeed that there was any contradiction or confusion in their stance. They staunchly refused, therefore, to entertain the idea that we might be purchased as we were but with a view to renegotiate, as it were downstream, once the newly configured PD services had embedded or not, with our 'new' commissioners. They did not accept that their suggestion that we change unilaterally (outside of a negotiation with future/would-be commissioners) represented a high-risk strategy. It was not, of course, of high risk to themselves who would soon be out of the frame. They seemed to be saying, in effect, 'Just change!' as if that would solve our problems and those of the wider PD system.

More unwelcome changes were to follow. It was, after all, the silly season of August, and in tune with this the Henderson Project Group, as if it were becoming too stable for its own good, metamorphosed into the aptly named 'Henderson Oversight Group'. (It was to last, in effect, only four months and to meet twice, but in that short passage of time would have two Chairs, the latter choosing to suspend its operation after its second meeting in October.) At its first meeting – its inauguration in August – it was stated, by the person leading on commissioning (the second to have been delegated to that role but the third actual incumbent) that, following receipt of some simple activity data from Henderson, i.e. by the end of September, we would have a decision regarding London's commissioning stance in relation to Henderson.

Well, September came and went, as is its wont. Another change of senior commissioning personnel in the system had meant that another 'Chair' had departed and so no decision was forthcoming. However, there was leaked 'news' in early October (via the third 'lead'). This stated that everything was on track for a positive outcome from London and also (following informal meetings and discussions between this third lead and Eastern and Southern Regions' commissioning colleagues) that these regions would very likely also be on board with commissioning a steady state for Henderson (i.e. at least till April 2007 – maybe even beyond, with some form of a three-year rolling contract!).

This was welcome news indeed, not least since being without our Director of Planning we felt vulnerable, knowing how we had fared in the past when as clinicians we were left to deal directly with commissioners, as members of our Steering Group. There remained much to do on the work that we had agreed to undertake for the commissioners in relation to detailed information about Henderson's service. A 10-page leaflet and a 60-page booklet were duly produced, under the excellent direction of the external consultant who now was working more with our Trust (but still kind of working with/for the commissioners). In the process we needed to re-present Henderson's activity by PCT – all 128 of them – which was duly done. It was therefore dismaying to learn in the second (October) meeting of the Oversight Group that not only had no decisions from London been taken (for the reasons stated above) but also that no guarantee of any decision from London could be given ahead of its forthcoming November meeting. My challenge that things had actually gone backwards was not well received! I tried harder (and louder) to clarify if I had misunderstood. What had happened to put matters in reverse? I asked. What of the positive tidings leaked to us by the third lead? I enquired. The collective indecision of the commissioners, I suggested, was already having an effect on Henderson's morale and staff retention and recruitment, since all staff knew we had no definite future beyond March 2006. According to local commissioners, adding to the problem was the fact that NSCAG would not/could not decide how it was to devolve its funding to PCTs, and without this it would be harder for PCTs to come to any agreement collectively. I failed to obtain a satisfactory answer to my request to the NSCAG member in the room to be updated on the reasons for a lack of progress on this matter since August. It seemed as if Henderson had to answer the commissioners' questions but not vice versa. This did not seem fair.

The PCTs could not therefore say 'yes' or 'no' to that which was not clearly offered to them. We were now informed there was to be a pan-London PD strategy that would be discussed. What, we wondered, might be the effect of this on Henderson's re-commissioning? Would matters have to wait, as we had been told previously that they would have to, until there was an agreed London strategy for PD? Such a wait – for who knew how long? – could be tantamount to closing us down, since it would be highly likely that more and more staff would leave (some were already planning to do so), and recruitment of suitably qualified highly specialised staff could be well-nigh impossible. 'Fiddling' and 'burning' in southern Italy came to mind.

My frustrated attempts to convey the urgency of the situation seemed only to identify me as unreasonable and petulant. The 'Oversight' meeting ended unhappily and the Chair, who announced that she wished she had cancelled the meeting beforehand, decided it would not be fruitful for it to be reconvened. Why not? Had it achieved its purpose? Had the purpose been to find a way to opt out of commissioning Henderson? At the time of writing we await the outcome of the postponed September agenda and to see if we have a decision, any decision, ahead of the arrival of a London PD strategy. Interestingly, the 'third lead' contacted me via email to ask if the independent replication research findings could be made available to him! I indicated that NSCAG were in the process of meeting with the independent scientists to review these and suggested he obtained an invitation to that meeting. (He made no mention of the meeting concerning Henderson's future, which by then had taken place – unless it had been cancelled. Obviously my worries about the service had fallen on deaf ears.) Eventually we heard, two weeks after their meeting (23 November), that we had London's PCT support until April 2007 but with certain caveats – as much as we could have hoped for at this time, though nowhere near sufficient. The optimism with which we had received this news the first time around was not present.

Conclusions

'Too many cooks spoil the broth' might pithily translate as 'Rapid turnover of commissioners/managers undermines the completion of complex (clinician-led) service innovation'! This theme runs through this book, like a river in flood washing away all in its path. This image might also be applicable to other problems that exist, more widely, in the NHS. Many parties seem to be legitimately involved in a project, such as replicating Henderson, and, to an extent, necessarily so. However, the more there are, the less likely it is that all are able to blend satisfactorily. Add to this unsatisfactory mix the relatively rapid turnover of many in management and other strategic positions, and the likelihood of any but the simplest and most local recipes being followed successfully, and the resulting meal being fit for consumption, is vanishingly small.

With the Henderson replication, all the cooks must bear some responsibility for their culinary creations – delectable or inedible as they turned out to be. Crucially, these cooks were: NSCAG, the three (or more) participating Trusts (Chief Executive/Medical Directors), the Steering Group, HDT and the staff and residents of the Henderson/HOST/Main House/Bridge House and Webb House. Too often it was not clear which cook was in charge of which stage of the recipe. This was especially pertinent when things started to go wrong. As a consequence, it took much longer than was helpful to rectify. Indeed, under such difficult circumstances, some cooks tended to turn the heat up while others rushed to remove the heated offering from the hob. Once on the table some thought the product to be edible, others delectable. Some found it unfit for human consumption. Which chef is to be believed?

CHAPTER EIGHT

To Future Chefs

Introduction

Even with hindsight, it may not always be possible to be sure that what one did was clearly right or wrong. One's power and control over events is often disappointingly small, and the number of events that can influence outcome in a project such as that described in this book is large. At a given point, even if it were possible to know that one had made the right decision, there could be many subsequent influences in the fullness of time, some quite unpredictable, that could undo or significantly modify the desired and intended outcome. In effect, these influences could be sufficient to nullify the correctness of the original decision, rendering a 'right' decision 'wrong' and vice versa!

We like to believe that we can learn from our experience. So, assuming that we can and that we can ascribe 'right' or ' wrong' to the decisions and courses of action (or inaction) taken or not taken, I shall endeavour to identify lessons that might be learned from my/our experiences of setting up services in the NHS. Obviously, I believe that there is more to be learned from what I now consider as having been 'wrong'. My hope therefore is that in describing our mistakes, others might be able to avoid them. This applies especially to any embarking or already embarked upon a similar endeavour to that described here. There are also those in positions of management, whose action (and inaction) might also affect the progress of these would-be NHS innovators, who might learn from what follows.

Contractual matters

The small print

I think that we should have tried harder to get clarity on the small print of the contract with NSCAG. In our defence, we had got worn down by what we experienced as the latter's unreasonable demands. They had required us to work and re-work the original bid, even to the tune of calculating the logistics for a service development that did not meet NSCAG's own stated requirements from us – to have a service that covered the whole country. The effect of this extra work (being in addition to that of our 'day jobs') distracted us from itemising aspects of the bid that later became contentious – in particular research and training. It proved to be a costly error that we did not get all the ingredients of our service listed at the first service level agreement. Nobody these days expects a steady-state situation to exist in the NHS for very long. But it had been a mistake to assume, just because there was nothing said or written to the contrary, that our statement of the originally submitted requirements would stand as the contract. The DH, no doubt, reserved the right to vary the conditions due to unforeseen circumstances. And there were plenty of circumstances to follow, whether or not unforeseen.

It is still a source of resentment to me personally that we had the whole research force axed during the course of the replication. This ruined the original plan (hatched with senior DH advisers) to triple Henderson's PD research capacity. This would have enabled us, potentially, to have been much more efficient in answering at least certain PD- and TC-related research questions. Without a dedicated research resource we could not so easily evaluate changes to one service in relation to the other two that would enable us to understand so much more about the process of how the TC worked. My personal research plans also lay in tatters as a result.

So the lesson is to get as much detail as possible into a contract before starting, as if doing business with a firm outside of the NHS, even if this causes delays to the enterprise in question. We were a mixture of too hasty, too naïve and too tired to bother with this, and we regretted it. The doing of it would not have guaranteed a different ultimate outcome but would probably have produced a different tone to the negotiations had NSCAG had to admit that they were varying the original contractual terms – as we saw it, moving the goalposts.

Rules of engagement and roles

Some of the lessons described in this section also apply in and overlap with many others in this chapter. With the high turnover of personnel in NSCAG and the three participating NHS Trusts, it would have helped that small number of us struggling consistently during the entire course of the project to have had more detail about what was agreed (and what was not) actually spelled out in writing. At least, I believe it to be so. I imagine then that we would not have encountered what we experienced as changes of direction and 'moving of goalposts', without justification or apology. This might not have changed the actual course taken by the project, since time does not stand still, even when the nature of the project is the modelling of a complex and dynamic institution for others to copy. However, the attitudes and the 'spirit' in which the replication was carried out would have been different – better.

It would probably have been preferable to identify how obstacles were to be overcome and by whom, related to the point about carrying out a financial 'risk assessment'. There are many places where this would have helped: disagreements within the Steering Group with respect to important decisions; financial resourcing in relation to NSCAG; service development problems in relation to individual

Trusts; clinical governance in relation to both NSCAG Trusts. Again, problems would not have been avoided wholesale but their resolution would have been made easier and smoother if we had envisaged a mechanism and planned ahead of time – forewarned would have been forearmed. Much of it could have been less adversarial.

Money and resources

Probity

Time and again the whole project's future was jeopardised by wrangling over money – not a surprise. Being so close to the Treasury, since NSCAG money came directly from that source, both this project and NSCAG had to be 'squeaky clean' – not that any of us was trying to defraud! It seemed to me, however, that local Trust custom and practice did not always represent what the DH believed to be the case. Most notably, there was the issue of turning revenue into capital – so heinous a crime. We should have documented clearly the fact that we would not be applying for capital funding from any public–private partnership scheme, and should have stated what our plans were to raise such monies. It is staggering to me now, looking back, that it was not a requirement to have this aspect made crystal clear at the outset by all concerned. Remember, although no money was forth-coming until April 1998, and all the costs till then had to be borne by the local participating Trusts, some of the research exercise was under way from January 1998, and there was also some spend on salaries in relation to the first staff employed. All of this would have been wasted had we been unable to find suitable premises, due to problems identifying the capital. Nobody could have seriously thought that, without their being involved in any prior discussion, the Regional Outposts (see Chapter 5) were considered to be a reliable source of such funding. The whole edifice could have crumbled early, on this financial issue.

There would seem to be a learning point for a number of different stake-holders here. Mere clinicians, such as myself, should not trust that their local pay-masters will take the trouble to look in sufficient detail at a project that does not derive from their existing budgets. Those in positions of financial responsibility should trouble to consider such basics unless there is a 'game' to be played here with central Government that I do not understand. Those involved centrally in initiating projects that have Ministerial backing would do well to ensure that the capital funding is taken care of. In the case of service innovation, especially of specialist services in places where there have been none, it should be clearly estab-lished how premises are to be identified and, if necessary, also how rendered fit for purpose. As has been seen (Chapter 5), even after the 'suitable' premises were found there was a considerable extra (refurbishment) expense to be met.

Realistic resources from the outset

Getting the right resources in place is about setting aside enough time to think and plan. Yet it is impossible to know in advance exactly what will be required. One solution might be to think of a number and double it! We had attended insufficiently to the risk that things could go wrong and thus often had not made appropriate contingency plans. Such planning aspects are now relatively commonplace in the NHS; however, at the time we started (1996) such thinking was not prevalent and none ever cautioned us in that direction, naïve as we were in matters of business.

Other than doubling the original estimate of the time needed, on the assumption that a lot of what could go wrong will go wrong, it is also worthwhile ensuring that all the necessary types of resources are considered – time, personnel, 'plant' and money. The last of these is clearly crucial, since it buys the others, at least it does so in large measure. Yet this is often the most difficult to calculate, since in the bidding situation a balance has to be struck between the absolutely necessary and the ideal. Competition tends to favour the cheaper bids. However, apart from the 'revenue-to-capital' debacle and niggling discussions around carrying over unspent money to the next financial year (vital to our project), this project did not suffer from financial under-resourcing. Yes, we could argue about funding for the research and training functions, but we have done so elsewhere.

We had not left enough time to obtain premises or to negotiate the NHS bureaucracy and I do not believe that more personnel (hence more money) would have helped much, if at all. NHS bureaucracy represents a formidable obstacle to innovation, which on account of the organisational units that comprise the NHS and the rules that apply, is unlikely ever to disappear. Future public–private initiatives might improve matters. For the time being, it would be important to factor in much more time and to create a more clearly 'phased' project design, with attendant costings, than we did. To do so, however, would have prolonged the expected time-scale of our project, thereby making it potentially more expensive, hence a less attractive and competitive bid. It feels, looking back, as if it were the organisation of our resources rather than its amount that was sub-optimal, and the lessons to be learned stem from this conclusion, which is not to diminish the need to obtain adequate resources, without which any project is doomed.

Meeting and managing

Communication

It would have helped all of us had the three participating Trusts, at the outset, established a programme of face-to-face meetings with NSCAG, to report back on the schedule of work and to revise 'rules' relating to the project and its operation, as necessary. Our progress was so slow to start with, and NSCAG had so few resources, that it did not occur to either side that there might be such a need. But to innovate services requires close relationships and mutual sensitivity between funders and funded, more so than we enjoyed. From NSCAG's side, I guess (in danger here of sympathy), they could not have legitimated putting in additional resource because the extra work to begin with was so slight. However, had they done so, this might have avoided any later embarrassment that could have followed if the whole project had failed.

We might have established how best to contact one another and how not to. Negative or other unwanted or unexpected contact can serve to sour relationships. Agreeing in advance who could call meetings or initiate communication and about what would have made life more congenial, if not necessarily more successful ultimately. The journey could have been more fun, if the driving conditions had been better. Both sides probably should own some responsibility for things turning out the way they did, which to my mind was sub-optimal.

Similar issues applied to an extent among the three participating Trusts and their respective personnel. The Steering Group, Replication Meetings and HDT had overlapping membership, and we had thought that good communication would emerge inevitably from such a structure. We believed that it had been crucial to attend to communication, since we were so dispersed geographically and would not have the luxury of casual or informal meetings that might 'oil the wheels' and allow the project to run smoothly. At the start, this plan appeared to work since there was only the Steering Group. As time progressed, however, two factors came increasingly into play. Internally, the nature of the Steering Group business increased to include that of running clinical services, as opposed to simply spending money, for example on purchasing premises and refurbishment. Then it was not always clear which forum was the right one in which to discuss issues to do with replication, which had a claim on all forums – Steering Group, Replication and HDT (an extended version incorporating the clinical leads from the two new services).

Externally, in relation to NSCAG, it was not always clear who we were, since sometimes we were the deputies of senior Trust personnel and at other times – confusingly in the same meeting – were our clinical selves. In a sense we then became both the 'managers' and the 'managed'. Any concerns that NSCAG had they took up with 'us'. Foolishly, we generally tried to respond to these, which only fuelled the idea that we were the appropriate body. It would probably have helped us if we could have taken stock at the point that these changes had taken place, and discussed whether we needed a different structure or membership for the Steering Group. In any case, we should probably have reiterated the structure to all concerned with the three Trusts so that they might have sanctioned or not our carrying on with it. No doubt internal Trust business and Trust mergers, etc. meant that our project was not often top of their list of priorities.

My belief now is that we had conflated two hierarchical levels (manager and managed) in the single body of the Steering Group, and that succeeding NSCAG representatives would treat us at times as if we were senior Trust management and would be disappointed by our responses. It would have been better if we (as Directors of the clinical services) had not been in direct communication with them unless there had been some express detail of clinical care that required a dialogue between commissioners and clinicians. I now appreciate that commissioners are entitled to be part of negotiations about the nature of services provided, hence a dialogue with clinicians might well have been appropriate at times. Even if this state of affairs were not entirely the responsibility of the Steering Group, we certainly ought to own up to a share of it.

Leadership, the delegation of authority and deputies

Leadership always sounds to me like a simple and straightforward idea. In one sense, I was the leader of this project, as Chair of the Steering Group. However, often I did not really have the necessary power to fulfil such a role. As discussed elsewhere, it felt frequently as if the real leaders resided in the Department of Health, within NSCAG to be precise. The lack of regular contact with them, however, made them 'back-seat drivers'. They could certainly operate the brake, one which none on the service provider side could release. But then NSCAG were not really leading, other than in the sense of defining the general direction of travel. The precise route down which to go – a mixture of both strategic and executive matters – was left to the Steering Group to decide, most of the time. NSCAG had made it clear to us, at least at the outset, that they wanted as little direct involvement as possible, given their slender resources at that time.

It was not sufficiently clear what power had been delegated to the Steering Group, either by NSCAG or, more particularly, by the three participating Trusts. We had thought that the success of our bid, which had outlined our plans and the establishment of a Steering Group, served to hand us sufficient power to deliver the project. This was naïve. The signatories of the bid were the Chief Executives. However, none of these could spare much time or real consideration to either strategic or operational issues concerning this replication project. Nominally, they were all members of the Steering Group led by me. How much they thought about this or were acutely aware that this was so, I do not know. Certainly those Chief Executives who merely inherited the project might be excused for having little interest, save when things went wrong or appeared to pose an unacceptably high risk of whatever sort. Yet they were full members, even if they regularly sent deputies. A similar state of affairs pertained to their respective Medical Directors.

Perhaps I was leading this group of high-ranking Trust personnel from three separate NHS Trusts. However, with hindsight I would have to say 'Well, sort of '. As long as things progressed without obvious difficulty or impediment, there was the illusion that I was leading. As a group, we had indeed confronted the issue of leadership early on. That had been a tricky but probably necessary stage in the cohering of the Steering Group. When inevitably the project ran into difficulties, however, it became clear just where the power-base actually lay – well, more or less clear – and where it did not. The prime example was that of the National Service Management Group, which attempted to form itself out of the ashes of the Steering Group but which failed to wrest any real authority from our respective Trusts. NSCAG increasingly realised they could work around this body by going directly to the Chief Executives and they demonstrated that they could do what the Steering Group had failed to do throughout its six years' life-span, i.e. to get the three Chief Executives in a room together. Sadly, this was in the terminal phase of the project and in relation to the NIMHE document that many of us thought would help to secure our futures. Another example was when it came to NSCAG's decision to decommission. At this point, those of us who had staffed the Steering Group and attempted to manage the single national PD service were totally sidelined. The Trusts were in sole charge, and clinicians were then completely excluded from all direct discussions and negotiations with NSCAG.

It might have helped to have had a member of the Trust Board, from one of the three Trusts, to lead the overall project. At times this would have meant that those in formal positions of management authority within the Trusts would have been the first people to speak to NSCAG, instead of those of us (clinicians) deputising. Having a senior Trust figurehead would also have kept up (or would have helped to keep up) the profile of the project through the rocky period of merger, one Trust with another. Such seniority in leadership would have made it easier to liaise with the new seniors involved in the reshuffles of staff at the highest levels. Such a leader might well have had greater success than I had with getting the three Chief Executives into the same room. A non-clinician Trust Board member, or perhaps a Medical Director, would have been in a stronger position to lead than was I.

Distances to travel

I have yet to calculate how far I travelled in the course of the entire replication project. Perhaps I never will. Maybe I do not really want to know. The fact of the matter is, however, that very many people, in the course of this whole enterprise, travelled many, many miles. The fact that much of this was by train means that it was an expensive endeavour, but then the clients we were attempting to benefit by extending our specialist service were known to be expensive to treat. The inclement weather did not help, nor did the appalling state of the rail network. Ours was a labour-intensive method, but then we believed at the time this development was called for, and I still hold to this. However, a different model of HDT (as discussed elsewhere in this chapter) might not only have helped to identify a better uptake of learning but might also have necessitated fewer visits, hence less travel and lower costs. It might have been, had we been aiming to communicate solely with the most senior staff, that we could have done so via video-conferencing – something we in fact experimented with towards the end of the project, in relation to management meetings.

Part of the original problem we were attempting to solve by this project was that vast areas of the country were poorly served. As with other disciplines there was some truth to the notion that London was best-served with services for people with severe PD. It seemed that showing willingness to travel might take away some of the elitist tag from Henderson (and London). I do believe that our efforts in bearing the brunt of the travel, especially in respect of the HDT membership, were appreciated. I hope that it was more appreciated than would have been our plugging in to a video camera! Face-to-face meetings should ideally make communication more authentic and effective, especially where the nature of the business is complex, sensitive or expensive.

There is no doubt that with the long distances involved more could and did go wrong, which meant, for example, that a lot of the potential HDT energy was dissipated. I am also in little doubt about the fact that Henderson's service felt stressed by the strain emanating from so many of its senior staff being away so often and for so long. Clearly, the same number of meetings, had they been much closer, would have been accommodated with much less disruption. (Interestingly, the average bed occupancy/length of stay figures over the period – often taken as markers of the health of a TC – did not appear to be unduly affected.) No doubt much would have been simpler if the new services had been closer to us, though replication even over short distances is not inevitably successful.

In the end there had to be a balance struck between face-to-face and distant communication, i.e. telephone, video-conferencing, etc. Where the nature of the business is the replication of a complex human system of organisation, it is hard to think other than that at least some face-to-face talking is indispensable. As the project developed over time and as familiarity and trust increased, it was easier to rely on distance communication. Sadly, however, at the most difficult point, leading up to the closure of Webb House, communication of any kind all but died out.

Shared concepts
The nature of the task

Early on, we were bamboozled by the structure/culture debate (later also taken up by the organisational researcher, as the 'spirit/letter problem' – see Chapter 6). Perhaps it had been inevitable that this would become our preoccupation. Replication was indeed the name of the game, so being able adequately to define it was crucial. We were concerned, however, since the process was being independently researched, that the decisive factors about whether replication had been achieved (or not) might be structural aspects of the services, i.e. those that were more readily measurable, such as the presence of a daily community meeting. We were faced with the need to identify those of Henderson's myriad structures that were necessary and those merely desirable or even redundant for the present purposes. (Later we considered 'tight' and 'loose' structures in relation to streamlining the national service.) There were no easy answers, since it is not possible to unravel a TC and identify its vital ingredients. The TC is not amenable to such deconstruction, except in imagination. The whole is greater than the sum of its parts (see Norton 2003). So even answering the structural question was problematic. We did not know precisely what structures needed to be replicated.

We all agreed that really it was the 'culture' which was the essential aspect to replicate, though knew that this was harder to define and harder to ascertain if it were present. It would after all not only need to reside in staff members but in the residents and, more than this, in the overarching staff team functioning (as well as that of the residents) and that of the whole TC. HDT had a similar task to that of the independent researchers, though utilising a very different methodology with which to deliver. HDT's attempt to re-define TC-relevant ideological statements as core behaviours was only partially successful. There was little enthusiasm for 'manualising'. Partly, this was because such an approach might have removed vital spontaneity from the system (and hence eradicated or prevented that which we needed to create). Partly, such an undertaking was felt to be impossibly large to achieve. My fear was that agreeing to replicate only the culture would leave us vulnerable to misunderstanding by the independent organisational researcher and might also spell an overall failure to achieve what we had set out to.

In the early stages, I was not convinced that all of us in the Steering Group held similar values or could suspend our own personal values in order to sign up to a shared set for the benefit of this project. Early disagreements, for example over the appointment procedure for the Director post, made it hard to feel certain that we held sufficient that was similar and pertinent to this collaborative venture. It might have been that having to 'copy', which the word 'replication' might imply, was unpalatable to those tasked with the copying. It did seem to be the best word we could find at the time, and we had not felt particularly exercised by the term at the outset. In being the 'copied' and not the 'copier', Henderson and I had the easier ride. But I also carried, perhaps unwisely and at times unhelpfully, the weight of responsibility for the research as Principal Investigator. Had we been able to adopt a more flexible concept or image than 'replication' we might, paradoxically, all have got on better together with a clearer shared vision of what it was that we had agreed to do. 'Innovation diffusion' may have conveyed a more liberal and creative spirit, and it relates to a body of literature, but it had been quite unfamiliar to most of us in the Steering Group. Understanding this process from an academic perspective could have helped us, as could thinking about the replication of 'processes' or of 'ways of knowing'. The notions we had in mind were too concrete, which was embarrassing, especially for those of us who were also dynamic psychotherapists!

Finally, we had been preoccupied with the translation of the Henderson into the new territories largely in terms of the clinical programme and were in danger of thinking that this was the sum total of the replication brief. Fortunately, we remembered, just in time (on Salford's unforgettably sunny day) that our brief needed to extend to much of the administration and some of the management structures. As it was to turn out, some of these aspects appeared to be crucial. First and foremost was the position of the TCs in respect of their respective Trust's management hierarchies, hence in relation to their power to identify sufficient managerial and administrative resource for the smooth pursuit of the project. As clinicians, we had perhaps devalued the role and importance of our managerial and administrative colleagues. Gaining greater agreement about what it was we were trying to replicate in such non-clinical domains should have enjoyed a high priority.

The HDT role

It seemed that I had under-estimated the complexity of the task, if not also the fact of human nature – another cardinal sin for a self-respecting and card-carrying psychotherapist. On the face of it, HDT simply had responsibility for setting up a training programme and we had been wise to do this with help (see Chapter 2). More than this, however, as part of facilitating 'on the job learning', we had had to identify when significant departures from the Henderson methods and attitudes had occurred. It was in the pursuit of this task that most confusion would surface, and we found that we did not all share the same concept of HDT's role. Some difficulties we had anticipated. We had tried, for example, to plan for there being resistance to learning. We had therefore, after discussion with the two new services, arrived at a position whereby HDT was to provide primarily 'support'. We were to be facilitative rather than corrective. Also the use of service users – the Volunteers – well versed in the methods of Henderson, we saw as potentially removing obstacles to learning that might come about from seeing HDT as comprising visiting (critical) experts. The Volunteers were also there to help with the assimilation, by the new services' residents, of the requisite attitudes and skills with which to gain most benefit from the TC approach. Using a range of disciplines within the HDT was also a cunning ruse to make the uptake of knowledge and skills almost irresistible – or so we had imagined!

It might have been more natural for HDT to have done business only through the more senior staff in the new services. They might have appreciated this, although, interestingly, none ever suggested that the HDT stop its visits or radically re-shape its processes. HDT could have comprised the same personnel (multi-disciplinary and Volunteers), but meet to hear of the seniors' concerns or about other matters that they might have chosen for discussion. This would undoubtedly have supported them in their positions of seniority and also allowed them to have been the ones to 'correct' any deviations from the Henderson model that might have derived from such a format. Alternatively, HDT might have visited as planned but not fed back to other than the senior staff, either at the time or later via Replication Meetings. Issues emanating could then have been discussed, with the potential benefits described above but also with the additional one of HDT having seen for themselves what was actually going on in this replication experiment. The main disadvantage that might have followed would have been the marginalising of front-line staff. However, this might have been preferable to reinforcing a senior/junior staff split, particularly as we observed in Birmingham. We do not know the truth of the matter, nor why, if we had played such a 'splitting' role, this had not been repeated in Crewe. Certainly, HDT felt itself to be caught up in 'splitting' processes, and this aspect might have been mitigated to an extent by utilising a different strategy from that chosen. As a result, it might have been easier to agree and maintain a shared view of the purpose of the HDT role and the methods chosen to effect this.

Across and within Trusts

'Reality' of cross-Trust structures

The Steering Group was a cross-Trust structure – involving personnel from all three Trusts – and invested with at least some authority to plan and spend NSCAG's money. Its legitimacy and power hailed from the fact that there was no other grouping tasked to do the particular business of replication. This meant that we could set up subgroups of the Steering Group, for example, in relation to research or training, which could also be both efficient and effective. In fact, various cross-Trust structures were envisaged and indeed were real enough to have borne fruit. Although generating little of its own new work, in the limited time available, the Research Group supported the successful completion of the independent research (see Chapter 6) in part due to the direction given it from Henderson's research hub (and in particular Dr Fiona Warren). Training too was another area, beyond that of HDT, which seemed destined to go places. An imaginative training scheme was fully worked out with collaboration from all three Trusts. The project was under the leadership of Chris Scanlon, the Henderson training lead. The success of these ventures reflected the 'reality' of their respective structures. The surrounding systems recognised them and did business with them (Manning 1980). A three-way partnership – not without considerable teething problems – truly emerged.

When it came to our capacity to set ourselves up as a cross-Trust 'National Service Management Group' (NSMG), however, we signally failed. It was as if delegated authority stopped at the stroke of the end of the development of the national service. Henceforth, the running of it would be via the three Trusts – in fact, this was the original vision of producing three autonomous services. It was only later that we had planned for the development of the NSMG. This would have been more powerful than our local management groups within the three participating Trusts. The NSMG might have helped us to argue their respective corners, and for this not to be seen as 'special pleading' but as a request for respect and tolerance of the exigencies of working the democratic TC model. When we eventually attempted to get formal recognition of this grouping, it became clear that it had no status. None within the three Trusts would accept it as having a separate validity. It was thus clear that, although we remained a national service, we were each, first and foremost, under local control. Local factors in management, clinical governance and human resources would come first.

Events, especially the various Trust mergers affecting/afflicting this project, played a role in undermining the authority actually invested in the structures we had set up. However, our need for authorisation varied according to the phase of the project. We had not anticipated sufficiently the effect of project milestones in altering the requirements of the structures we had set up. With hindsight, we should perhaps have celebrated each milestone, taking care to review the necessity for its continued existence. One such milestone was the opening of the two new units, another was the transition from setting up to 'established' units, 18 months post-opening. Some of these transitions had real-world meaning, for example, indicating the direction of flow of money from NSCAG, though others were subtler in their effect.

The lesson learned is to review the fitness of the structures – regular meetings or forums – for purpose, to make necessary changes and to present any new structural 'product', a forum of some sort, to all relevant parties, lest they cease to recognise and do business with them. Failure to do so might be rectifiable in the short term. However, chronic misuse or disuse probably spells the 'death' of a structure, with no possibility of resurrection (again see Manning 1980).

Local relations

This topic relates to that just discussed. What now seems to me elementary is the need to keep in touch with one's relevant Trust members about matters going on in a project such as the one described here. It is not sufficient to make assumptions that people either know or are interested to get to know what they need to know. With me, it was a matter of not thinking deeply enough, but also not wanting to bother the 'top brass' about a relatively lowly project – particularly at the time of other major business, namely that of merger.

The replication had started with a small number of us, when Henderson was part of a larger 'general' NHS Trust. Its Chief Executive delegated almost total responsibility for the Mental Health Service to a deputy with whom we had regular and close contact. As long as this pertained, all could be assured that necessary news would be swiftly transmitted and any necessary action taken (for example an 8 a.m. meeting of relevant parties to resolve the issue of the Director appointment in Birmingham). However, this successful situation changed as a job-share arrangement supervened for this crucial Mental Health leader. At times, it was the one and at other times the other 'half' who attended our meetings. In their own ways, both were able and committed to the project, yet inevitably this divisive arrangement detracted from the actual time each spent thinking and doing in relation to our project. Perhaps we should have argued to work simply with one or other party, rather than acquiescing with the plan!

The merger of our original Trust with a much larger was one heralded by a so-called 'steady state year' – during which transition period we endured five managers. This contrasted with the non-steady state of the previous seven years with only a single manager! And, within the new Trust, the seniority of our managers was much lower. Even when fully invested in the project, they would no longer carry such weight as in former days when our managers were able to inform, or be informed by, the most senior Trust levels. At a stroke we, the project, were downgraded. Arguably, the project at the time of the merger should have been independent of senior patronage, but events tell a different story.

It would have been wiser to have spent time updating the new Chief Executive and Trust Board on the nature and detail of our project or, at least, to have made an offer to do so. In not so doing, beyond an informal talk with the Chief Executive, in connection with the merger – apparently I had been, at the time, a relevant senior doctor to have on board – our project only became visible when running into choppy waters. 'We', the project, thus became synonymous with 'problems'. So, far from having unequivocal support, we had moved from being (relatively) the 'jewel in the crown' , within the old Trust, to a 'thorn in the side' of the new Trust – not a comfortable location. My complaint to the Chief Executive at the lack of a promised steady state and its damaging effect on our project was met with incredulity and annoyance. With hindsight, I can almost see matters from the Chief Executive's perspective, though not quite. Certainly, I should have been more energetic and proactive in promoting the project and thereby would have had a much better chance of obtaining support at an appropriate senior level, when needed.

This was a big project to undertake as (in my own case) a part-timer. Like me, my Director colleagues were also struggling to find mental space to consider the niceties of internal Trust personal relations, alongside the need to deliver their clinical services. However, these niceties are necessary in the modern NHS and particularly in the face of massive personnel change, as occurred via the moving on of Chief Executives and Trust mergers. Ideally, as the three Directors, we would have pooled our resources and made joint and regular presentations to the three Trust Boards, or at least offered to do so. It would then have been harder for the differing functions of Trust and clinical service, in relation to NSCAG, to have become conflated.

People

All aboard

In creating more 'Hendersons', there was clearly something in it for some of us, as well as a lot of extra work. For the majority of Henderson staff, however, there was precious little. The team had indeed been united in valuing the clinical work of the place and believing that there should be more such places, in the face of what we felt was an inadequate national resource for PD individuals. But the development of the other two services drained the 'parent' of some senior personnel, at least part-time. Also, being part-time (in relation to a programme such as Henderson's) meant also not being in the know sufficiently to contribute as previously, even when present. The sequestration of senior staff caused by the formation of the HDT thus represented a double loss to the team. Our absence meant that the gaps left needed to be filled by other seniors. In turn those 'below' would need to fill the gaps left by them. In short, none of the staff team would be unaffected. And the effect would be more, and harder, work, hence more stress and some would leave or in other ways fall by the wayside. Those involved in Henderson's Outreach also had something to lose by needing to take on a much larger catchment population in spite of only a small increase in resources. The effect of the replication was thus to create a relative shortfall there too.

Perhaps we should have toughed it out and waited for the negative forces of the 1990s NHS winds of change to blow themselves out. I believe now that we would have weathered the storm. However, the successful bid to NSCAG had been our third in three years, so it should not be under-estimated how insecure we felt – rightly or wrongly. The stress on the staff occasioned by the replication would have been less, I now believe, had I spent more time thinking through the implication for the whole staff team. This may not have meant any less work to do by the team, but the sense of shared ownership of the project would have been wider and the burden may have felt less heavy. Some staff who left, for one reason or another, during the development may not have done so.

Local histories and personalities

Our partnership to set up NHS services was not a marriage, certainly not one made in heaven. But, just as it is customary for prospective spouses to meet each other's respective families and friends to find out more about shared and different values, as well as much else, so it is probably wise to probe the recent and distant history of one's future collaborators. This we had done, to an extent. We felt we had chosen wisely. However, we did not know each other well or understand much of our respective family's histories or aspirations. As judged by the organisational researchers, these were to be potentially influential factors in the taking up of the diffused service innovation.

We had known of Birmingham's previous plans, for example, to develop inpatient services. But we may have under-estimated the extent of this ambition or that our project was really providing the 'means' for a quite different 'end' (see Birtle *et al.* 2004). In a sense, some writing had been on the wall, when the new Unit was named 'Main', after Tom Main, progenitor of a different treatment model to that of the Henderson! (We at Henderson continue to value the perceptive and persuasive writings of Tom Main, however, and his contributions to the thinking about the TC's cultural essence: see Main 1983; Norton 1992). The Salford collaboration, of course, had appropriated some Henderson personnel to be their 'local' personalities. Although this was probably a sensible step for them to take, it was not one which was particularly welcomed by Henderson; to an extent it represented an alternative method of TC model dissemination. Our overt and agreed model was not to transport staff to reside in distant places and to develop a new service *in situ* – 'theirs' was at variance with 'our' model.

Inevitably the personalities of the three Directors contributed to rivalries, which did not always deliver a speedy or correct analysis and appropriate action plan. Being, roughly, contemporaries probably fuelled a desire to out-perform one another in some way – consciously or unconsciously. All in all, however, my sense is that the spirit of collaboration was in the ascendancy and that, in spite of everything, even including the tragic closure of Webb House on 14 July 2004 – aged three and a half years – the result of this replication experiment was more success than failure. Mostly, I am proud of the venture. Posterity will be the ultimate judge of its success.

Appendix

NOTES OF THE EXTENDED REPLICATION MEETING
Walton Hall, Warwickshire, 11 and 12 December 2001

1. The purpose of the meeting was to acknowledge progress in establishing the two new bases and agree what form of organisation is necessary for running the three bases in their established form as a single national service.

2. Those present were:

Henderson/Sutton	Kingsley Norton, Harjinder Sehmi, Diana Menzies, Lawrence Higgens
Main House/Birmingham	Jan Birtle, Michael Bennett, Chris Newrith, Fiona McGroer
Webb House/Crewe	Keith Hyde, Michael Gopfert, Mary Lee, Amanda Weir
Researcher	Sue Ormrod
Facilitator	Andy Holder

The past two years

3. Each of the three bases plotted their positive and negative feelings (above and below a time line) over the past two years. There were two key issues:

   - The overall positive and improving sense of feeling of the two new bases compared to the Henderson – partly due to taking on new staff rather than losing staff, partly the challenge of the new compared to the on-going nature of the other; and partly extra demands on the Henderson.

   - The inevitable personal and base variations – due to new posts and hiccups in the building/development work.

4. The implications drawn were:

- There is a lot to celebrate individually and collectively – what has been achieved is no mean thing and it is the result of much effort and commitment over the period and before.

  Suggested action – there could be a joint celebration to mark the achievement.

- The need to support the Henderson, under pressure from lack of staff, in a reciprocal way to which it has supported others.

  Suggested action – there should be some clear task leads taken in the other bases for the whole service.

- The dynamics of feelings and work overload are critical for all the bases.

  Suggested action – development of a method for workload measurement and management could greatly help the impact on feelings and fatigue.

Headlining the next two years

5.   Each base was asked to create some headline achievements for the next two years. These could form the basis for a vision for each base and the common threads drawn together for the national service. The headlines were:

Henderson

- Integrated research
- Training and collaboration
- Full staff team
- Positive evaluation outcome
- Entry events
- Valued by the Trust
- Expansion and development of Outreach
- Blossoming umbrellas
- Improved built environment
- Secure funding

Main House

- Robust. Five stars from NSCAG
- Demand exceeds supply – ten new centres planned
- Core understanding in staff team (maturity) achieved – Eureka
- Valued both internally and externally

- Three in a bed sex romp!
- Warm glow reaches Henderson
- United! Psychotherapy and Social Therapy tie the knot

Webb House

- Consolidating the culture of the flattened hierarchy
- Developing, consolidating our relationship with the external world
- Clear roles and goals in all our activities
- More decision making by the staff and increasing confidence
- Training, training, supervision, training, training, supervision...
- Survive healthily and happily

Suggested action – each base to work these up with staff and merge into a specific one page statement with outcomes, identifying where issues need to be common across the national service.

Loose/Tight: Clinical Practice

6. The group sought to distil the tight – essentially common – characteristics of the service nationally. As a 'first take' they were:

Overall

- To provide a revolutionary and effective challenge to the medical model
- Each base to have residential and outreach services
- Each base to operate as a single team with two functions (for integration, development and resource decisions).

Referral/Selection

- Staff to screen consistently both in the way they apply the exclusion criteria (e.g. age, risk) and speak/communicate with referrers and potential users.
- Selection groups always to have a majority of residents.
- Information for the three bases is kept consistently and regularly shared on the profiles of those selected/not selected (e.g. gender, severity) for joint review of audit, development and risk patterns.

Residential

- The social therapy capacity is 24/7/365.

- Self-help and empowerment are the central values.

- A key strength is the capacity to muster the resources of the whole institution.

- The Top Three plus two duty staff is central modelling the capacity necessary for thinking, collaborating and empowering.

- There are a variety of meeting sizes having different functions with real power and responsibility.

- Continuity and coherence are provided in reviewing one day and planning the next by 'The Five'.

- There is always a culture of 'being held in mind'.

- All staff involved in groups attend after-groups.

- Key outcomes are length of stay and (logged) variety of responsibilities.

- Aims of treatment need to be spelt out more clearly e.g. relational and healthy dependency – Fairburn, Masterson, Benjamin.

- The role of staff needs to be spelt out more clearly in a self/other help process – the community as nurturer and doctor.

Outreach

- Review the labelling of this activity – it has data capture and resource implications. In particular the processes of comparability, learning and external presentation.

- Distinguishing the core/non-core funded elements is essential for identifying those that are good for training, marketing and referral and their resource aspects.

  Suggested action – a decision be made to work this up. How elaborately? when? and who? to be made clear.

Loose/Tight Organisational Characteristics

7. Three subgroups – the directors, clinical practitioners and administrators – then examined the organisational imperatives to back up the service nationally. The list of issues is set out in the Annexe. From this a series of 'must do' priorities (by March) were identified and the same groups worked them up into outline action plans. These topics are to be worked

up and reported upon by the 9th January – the next Replication Group meeting. The task groups are shaping up ideas and action for:

- Steering group mechanism – Jan, Keith, Kingsley
- Inclusion processes – Amanda, Harjinder, Fiona
- Common financial system – Mary, Lawrence, Michael B.

    Suggested action – groups to produce a note prior to the 9th January meeting outlining the issues and crucially, proposed action.

Follow-up

There was a general feeling that the meeting had highlighted some key characteristics that are important for the service if it is to operate at the national level. Notably these were the need:

- To have strong, single point of management of those things you hold in common (both clinically and administratively) – steering (managing) group (para 7);
- To recognise and respond to one another's particular pressures and feelings (para 4);
- For each base of direction, and collectively for all bases to draw together common strands of commitment e.g. training, research for an overall vision (para 5);
- To share a common understanding of the core/tight characteristics of the clinical practice that hold the three bases together (para 6);
- To agree a mechanism to monitor, research and review practice between the three bases;
- To agree priority tasks that need tackling and finishing (para 7);
- To agree divisions of labour that allow one base to lead for the others e.g. it was suggested that Webb lead on finance, Main House on clinical governance, and Henderson on research (?). There clearly could be many other functions which the overall managing/steering group could identify and negotiate delegations.

9. There has undoubtedly been much achieved at considerable effort. The future of this national service will rest upon active, mutual organisation and support. There seems to me to be a strong commitment to this despite some fatigue. A commitment to putting in place rapidly the priority building blocks of organisation together with trusting one another to get on with common tasks for the whole seems to offer much promise.

ANNEXE: ORGANISATIONAL TIGHT CHARACTERISTICS

Items *ed are regarded as 'must dos' by March 2002

Administrative Group

Structures

- Clear structure with terms of reference reporting to a 'steering' function
- Clear internal structures with understanding of the purpose and role of management and business group
- *Regular meetings of peers

Systems and mechanisms

- Consistent reporting for finance, activity, research, complaints, serious incidents etc (common measures)
- Shared policies and procedures
- Good reliable communications systems
- Consistent IT support systems

Roles and delegations

- *Understanding of 'who or which group' (steering and subgroups) has authority to make 'which' decisions (management group/business meeting/community meeting)
- Common frameworks for information (e.g. finance)
- Shared, timely, accurate information regularly reviewed by management groups

Information and data

- *Shared and consistent data sets – minimum to meet requirements
- *Common frameworks for information (e.g. finance as required internally, nationally, by Trusts and by NSCAG)

Culture and practice

- Everyone shares an appreciation of 'doing'
- Allowing yourself time to 'do' – balancing time in meetings with time to make things happen
- Identification of core role

References

Baron, C. (1987) *Asylum to Anarchy*. London: Free Association Books.

Becker, H., Geer, B., Hughes, E.C. and Strauss, A.L. (1977) *Boys in White*. Chicago, IL: Chicago University Press.

Birtle, J., Newrith, C., Brown, I., Mousse, B., Bennett, M. and Mackey, G. (2004) 'Leadership in a new therapeutic community: Learning to regulate the temperature.' *Therapeutic Communities 25*, 2, 85–99.

Briggs, D (2002) *A life well lived. Maxwell Jones: a memoir*. London: Jessica Kingsley Publishers.

Clark, P. (1987) *Anglo-American Innovation*. New York: De Gruyter.

Conte, H.R., Plut, R. and Karasu, T.B. (1980) 'A self-report borderline scale: discriminate validity and preliminary norms.' *Journal of Nervous and Mental Disease 168*, 428–435.

Czarniawska, J.B. (1997) *Narrating the Organisation*. London: University of Chicago Press.

Department of Health (2001) *Research governance framework for health and social care*. London: Department of Health.

Dolan, B.M. and Norton, K. (1992) 'One year after the NHS Bill: The extra-contractual referral system and Henderson Hospital.' *Psychiatric Bulletin 16*, 745–747.

Dolan, B.M. and Norton, K. (1998) 'Audit and survival: Specialist inpatient psychotherapy in the national health service.' In M. Patrick and R. Devanhill (eds) *Rethinking Clinical Audit: The Case of Psychotherapy Services in the NHS*. London: Routledge.

Erikson, E. (1956) 'The problem of ego identity.' *Journal of the American Psychoanalytical Association 4*, 56–121.

Fitzgerald, L., Ferlie, E., Wood, M. and Hawkings, C. (2002) 'Interlocking interactions: The diffusion of innovation in health care.' *Human Relations 55*, 12, 1429–1450.

Gabbard, G. (1986) 'The treatment of the 'special' patient in a psychoanalysis hospital.' *International Review of Psychoanalysis 13*, 333–347.

Hammersley, M. and Atkinson, P. (1995) *Ethnography* (Second Edition). London: Routledge.

Harrison, T. and Clark, D. (1992) 'The Northfield experiments.' *British Journal of Psychiatry 160*, 698–708.

Hatch, M. (1997) *Organisation Theory: Modern, Symbolic and Postmodern Perspectives*. Oxford: Oxford University Press.

Haugsgjerd, S. (1987) 'Toward a theory for milieu treatment of hospitalized borderline patients.' In J.S. Grotstein, M.F. Solomon and J.A. Lang (eds) *The Borderline Patient: Emerging Concepts in Diagnosis, Psychodynamics, and Treatment*. Mahwah, NJ: Lawrence Erlbaum Assoc.

Hinshelwood, R. (1988) 'Psychotherapy in an inpatient setting.' *Current Opinion in Psychiatry 1*, 304–308.

Holmes, J. (1999) 'Psychotherapeutic approaches to the management of severe personality disorder in general psychiatric settings.' *Psychiatric Bulletin 1*, 29–68.

Jones, M. (1952) *Social Psychiatry: A Study of Therapeutic Communities*. London: Tavistock.

Jones, M. (1979) *Social Psychiatry in Practice: The idea of the Therapeutic Community*. Harmondsworth: Penguin.

Kennard, D. (1989) 'The therapeutic impulse: What makes it grow?' *Therapeutic Communities 10*, 155–163.

Kennard, D. (1996) 1946: 'The papers that launched the therapeutic community – special commemorative issue.' *Therapeutic Communities 17*, 2.

Kernberg, O. (1986) *Severe Personality Disorders: Psychotherapeutic Strategies*. New Haven, CT: Yale University Press.

Kisely, S. (1999) 'Psychotherapy for severe personality disorder: Exploring the limits of evidence based purchasing. (comment).' *British Medical Journal 318*, 7195, 1410–1412.

Lambert, H. (1981) *Analysis, Repair and Individuation.* London: Academic Press.

Lewis, L.K. and Seibold, D.R. (1993) 'Innovation modification during intra-organisational adoption.' *Academy of Management Review 18,* 2, 322–354.

Main, T.F. (1946) 'The hospital as a therapeutic institution.' *Bulletin of the Menninger Clinic 10,* 66–68.

Main, T.F. (1983) 'The concept of the therapeutic community: Its variations and vicissitudes.' In M. Pines (ed) *The Evolution of Group Analysis.* London: Routledge and Kegan Paul.

Manning, N. (1980) 'Collective disturbance in institutions: A sociological view of crisis and collapse.' *Therapeutic Communities 1,* 147–158.

Manning, N. (1989) *The Therapeutic Community Movement: Charisma and Routinization.* London and New York: Routledge and Kegan Paul.

Manning, N., and Blake, R. (1979) 'Implementing ideals.' In R.D. Hinshelwood and N. Manning (eds) *Therapeutic Communities: Reflections and Progress.* London: Routledge and Kegan Paul.

Meek, L. (1988) 'Organisational culture: origins and weaknesses.' *Organisation Studies 9,* 4, 453–473.

Miller, L.J. (1989) 'Inpatient management of borderline personality disorder: A review and update.' *Journal of Personality Disorders 3,* 122–134.

NIMHE (2003) *Personality Disorder: No Longer a Diagnosis of Exclusion.* Policy implementation guidance for the development of services for people with personality disorder. London: Department of Health.

Norton, K. (1992) 'A culture of enquiry: Its preservation or loss.' *Therapeutic Communities 13,* 1, 3–26.

Norton, K. (1997a) 'In the prison of severe personality disorder.' *Journal of Forensic Psychiatry 8,* 2, 285–298.

Norton, K. (1997b) 'In-patient psychotherapy – Integrating the other 23 hours.' *Current Medical Literature – Psychiatry 8,* 2, 31–37.

Norton, K. (2003) 'Henderson Hospital: Greater than the sum of its sub-groups.' *Group Work 13,* 3, 65–100.

Norton, K., Healy, K. and Lousada, J. (2005) 'Specialist services in England: A case for managed clinical networks?' *Psychiatric Bulletin 29,* 365–368.

Ormrod, S. and Norton, K. (2003) 'Beyond tokenism in service user involvement: Lessons from a democratic therapeutic community replication project.' *Therapeutic Communities 24,* 105–114.

Rapoport, R. (1960) *The Community as Doctor.* London: Tavistock.

Reed, J. (1994) *Report of the Department of Health and Home Office Working Group on Psychopathic Disorder.* London: Department of Health and Home Office.

Roberts, J.P. (1980) 'Destructive processes in a therapeutic community.' *Therapeutic Communities 1,* 159–170.

Robertson, M., Swan, J. and Newell, S. (1996) The role of networks in the diffusion of technological innovation.' *Journal of Management Studies 33,* 3, 333–359.

Rogers, E. (1983) *Diffusion of Innovations* (Third Edition). New York: Free Press.

Rosen, M. (1991) 'Coming to terms with the field: understanding and doing organisational ethnography.' *Journal of Management Studies 28,* 1, 1–23.

Stacey, R. (2000) *Strategic Management and Organisational Dynamics.* Harlow: Financial Times/Prentice Hall.

Van de Ven, A., Polley, D., Garaud, R. and Venkataraman, S. (1999) *The Innovation Journey.* Oxford: Oxford University Press.

Weick, K.E. (1995) *Sensemaking in Organisations.* London: Sage.

Whiteley, J.S. (1978) 'The dilemmas of leadership in the therapeutic community and the large group.' *Group Analysis 11,* 40–47.

Whiteley, J.S. (1980) 'The Henderson Hospital: A community study.' *Therapeutic Communities 1,* 1, 38–57.

Whiteley, J.S. (1986) 'Sociotherapy and psychotherapy in the treatment of personality disorder. Discussion paper.' *Journal of the Royal Society of Medicine 79,* 721–725.

Whiteley, J.S. and Collis, M. (1987) 'The therapeutic factors in group psychotherapy applied to the therapeutic community.' *Therapeutic Communities 8,* 21–31.

Winnicott, D.W. (1972) 'The capacity to be alone.' In *The maturational processes and the facilitating environment.* London: The Hogarth Press and the Institute of Psycho-analysis.

Subject Index

Note: page numbers in *italics* refer to figures and tables

Author Index